ADVANCES IN

Pediatrics

Editor-in-Chief
Carol D. Berkowitz, MD, FAAP, FACEP

Chief, Division of General Pediatrics,
Department of Pediatrics Aurora,
Harbor-UCLA Medical Center,
Distinguished Professor of Pediatrics,
David Geffen School of Medicine at UCLA,
Torrance, California

ELSEVIER

PHILADELPHIA LONDON TORONTO MONTREAL SYDNEY TOKYO

ADVANCES IN
Pediatrics

VOLUMES 1 THROUGH 65 (OUT OF PRINT)

VOLUME 66

Publishing Director, Medical Reference: Dolores Meloni
Editor: Kerry Holland
Developmental Editor: Donald Mumford

Editorial Office:
Elsevier
1600 John F. Kennedy Blvd,
Suite 1800
Philadelphia, PA 19103-2899

International Standard Serial Number: 0065-3101
International Standard Book Number: 13: 978-0-323-72257-5

ADVANCES IN
Pediatrics

CONTRIBUTORS

EMILY J. ANKUS, BS, University of South Florida Morsani College of Medicine, Tampa, Florida

CAROL D. BERKOWITZ, MD, FAAP, FACEP, Chief, Division of General Pediatrics, Department of Pediatrics, Harbor-UCLA Medical Center, Distinguished Professor of Clinical Pediatrics, David Geffen School of Medicine at UCLA, Torrance, California

REBECCA C. BRADY, MD, Division of Infectious Diseases, Department of Pediatrics, Professor of Clinical Pediatrics, Cincinnati Children's Hospital Medical Center, University of Cincinnati College of Medicine, Cincinnati, Ohio

KATHERINE J. DEANS, MD, MHSc, Professor of Surgery, Department of Pediatric Surgery, Center for Surgical Outcomes Research, Nationwide Children's Hospital, Columbus, Ohio

CHARLENE DEKONENKO, MD, Surgical Scholar, Department of Surgery, Children's Mercy Kansas City, Kansas City, Missouri

ELISSA R. ENGEL, MD, Department of Pediatrics, University of South Florida Morsani College of Medicine, Tampa, Florida

CHRISTOPHER FERBER, MD, Chief Resident, Department of Pediatrics, Harbor-UCLA Medical Center, Torrance, California

RAYMOND FERNANDEZ, MD, Pediatric Neurology Associates, Director, Muscular Dystrophy Association Care Center, Shriners Hospital for Children, Tampa, Florida

HEATHER FORKEY, MD, Associate Professor of Pediatrics, Division Chief, Child Protection Program and Foster Children Evaluation Services (FaCES), Department of Pediatrics, UMass Memorial Children's Medical Center, University of Massachusetts Medical School, Worcester, Massachusetts

JASON D. FRASER, MD, Associate Professor, Department of Surgery, Children's Mercy Kansas City, School of Medicine, University of Missouri Kansas City, Kansas City, Missouri

MARIA GIERON-KORTHALS, MD, Department of Pediatrics, Division of Child Neurology, University of South Florida Morsani College of Medicine, Tampa, Florida

JESSICA GRIFFIN, PsyD, Associate Professor of Psychiatry and Pediatrics, Executive Director, Child Trauma Training Center, Department of Psychiatry, University of Massachusetts Medical School, Worcester, Massachusetts

WILLIAM HENNRIKUS, MD, Professor of Pediatric Orthopaedics, Penn State College of Medicine, Hershey, Pennsylvania

CATHERINE J. HERNANDEZ, MS, DNP Student, University of South Florida College of Nursing, Tampa, Florida

ALEXANDRA L. HOWARD, DO, MPH, Department of Pediatrics, University of South Florida Morsani College of Medicine, Tampa, Florida

MARCUS D. JARBOE, MD, Associate Professor, Section of Pediatric Surgery, Department of Surgery, Associate Professor, Division of Vascular and Interventional Radiology, Department of Radiology, University of Michigan, Mott Children's Hospital, Ann Arbor, Associate Professor

PAUL B. KAPLOWITZ, MD, PhD, Professor Emeritus, Division of Endocrinology, Children's National Hospital, George Washington University School of Medicine & Health Sciences, Washington, DC

AIMEE G. KIM, MD, Pediatric Surgery Critical Care Fellow, Section of Pediatric Surgery, Department of Surgery, University of Michigan, Mott Children's Hospital, Ann Arbor, Michigan

SHAUN M. KUNISAKI, MD, MSc, Associate Professor of Surgery, Associate Professor of Gynecology and Obstetrics, Division of General Pediatric Surgery, Johns Hopkins Children's Center, Johns Hopkins University, Johns Hopkins University School of Medicine, Baltimore, Maryland

AMY E. LAWRENCE, MD, Research Fellow, Department of Pediatric Surgery, Center for Surgical Outcomes Research, Nationwide Children's Hospital, Columbus, Ohio

CHARLES M. LEYS, MD, MSCI, Associate Professor of Surgery and Pediatrics, Chief, Division of Pediatric Surgery, University of Wisconsin School of Medicine and Public Health, American Family Children's Hospital, Madison, Wisconsin

KONSTANCE C. MACKIE, MS, LCDR, NC, USN, DNP Student, University of South Florida College of Nursing, Tampa, Florida

CATHERINE S. MAO, MD, Professor, Division of Endocrinology, Professor, Department of Pediatrics, David Geffen School of Medicine at UCLA, Harbor-UCLA Medical Center, The Lundquist Institute of Biomedical Innovation at Harbor-UCLA, Torrance, California

PETER C. MINNECI, MD, MHSc, Professor of Surgery, Department of Pediatric Surgery, Center for Surgical Outcomes Research, Nationwide Children's Hospital, Columbus, Ohio

VALERIE PANZARINO, MD, Associate Professor, Department of Pediatrics, University of South Florida, Tampa, Florida

JUAN FELIPE RICO, MD, Division of Hematology/Oncology, Department of Pediatrics, University of South Florida Morsani College of Medicine, Tampa, Florida

RYAN RIDENOUR, MD, Resident R4, Penn State College of Medicine, Hershey, Pennsylvania

PHILIP ROSENTHAL, MD, Professor of Pediatrics, Department of Pediatric Gastroenterology, Hepatology, and Nutrition, University of California, San Francisco, San Francisco, California

ALICIA GILL ROSSITER, DNP, Lt Col (Retired) USAFR NC, Associate Professor, University of South Florida College of Nursing, Tampa, Florida

SARA KATHRYN SMITH, MD, Assistant Professor of Pediatrics, Department of Pediatric Gastroenterology, Hepatology, and Nutrition, University of California, San Francisco, San Francisco, California

SASHA SVENDSEN, MD, Assistant Professor of Pediatrics, Child Abuse Pediatrician, Child Protection Program and Foster Children Evaluation Services (FaCES), Department of Pediatrics, UMass Memorial Children's Medical Center, University of Massachusetts Medical School, Worcester, Massachusetts

JENNIFER K. YEE, MD, Associate Professor, Division of Endocrinology, Associate Professor, Department of Pediatrics, David Geffen School of Medicine at UCLA, Harbor UCLA Medical Center; The Lundquist Institute of Biomedical Innovation at Harbor-UCLA, Torrance, California

CONTENTS VOLUME 67 • 2020

New Developments in Diagnosis, Treatment, and Management of Duchenne Muscular Dystrophy

Maria Gieron-Korthals and Raymond Fernandez

Advances in Pediatrics 67 (2020) xix–xx
ADVANCES IN PEDIATRICS

Introduction

Carol D. Berkowitz, MD, FAAP, FACEP

Certainly 2020 turned out NOT to be the year many of us thought it would be. The date suggested visual acuity and a bright future, but it turned out to be the opposite, with images of masks, staggering statistics of deaths, the pervasive admonition to "socially distance," and a sense of loneliness and isolation. None of this was on our radar screen in the spring of 2019 as we put together the 67th issue of *Advances in Pediatrics* updates and reviews on the challenging topics facing pediatricians. Fortunately, as we go to press in the spring of 2020, things seem to be improving, and the needs of children, beyond COVID-19, still need to be addressed. As in the past, the 2020 issue of *Advances in Pediatrics* covers the whole gamut of pediatrics. Assessing the social determinants of health, toxic stress, and adverse childhood experiences continues to be emphasized as critical to a child's full medical evaluation. An underaddressed pediatric population are military-connected children and their unique needs, especially when they are cared for in civilian primary care settings. While these children are particularly vulnerable because of frequent moves and parental absences, all children can benefit from pediatric advice to caregivers about fostering strong attachments (the foundation of childhood resilience) and teaching positive parenting principles. And while COVID-19 became the infectious disease "du jour" with concerns about transmissibility, high mortality, the paucity of proven treatments, and the lack of a vaccine, we need to celebrate the remarkable progress made in addressing other infectious diseases, such as meningococcal infections and hepatitis C. Newer vaccines against *Neisseria meningitidis* have resulted in a dramatic decrease in the incidence of the disease in the United States. Similarly, the development of oral direct-acting antivirals has improved the management of hepatitis C in the pediatric population. Equally dramatic progress has been made in the management of sickle cell disease with the development of newer Food and Drug Administration–approved medications (L-glutamine, crizanlizumab-tmca, and voxelator) and the prospect of bone marrow transplantation and gene therapy. Of late, there has been a lot of interest in type 2 diabetes and its increased emergence in the pediatric population, particularly those who are obese. Importantly, there have been significant changes in the management of type 1 diabetes in children, including advancements in pump technology, continuous glucose monitoring, and "closed loop" insulin pump systems, which have revolutionized treatment. Changes in the age of puberty have also been recognized

https://doi.org/10.1016/j.yapd.2020.05.001
0065-3101/20/© 2020 Published by Elsevier Inc.

with both boys and girls entering puberty at an earlier age, placing an additional challenge on recognizing when development is precocious or simply a variation of normal. It is critical to make this distinction and not implement very expensive therapy to stop what may be normal pubertal progression. Urolithiasis, often thought of as an adult disorder, can also affect children. The condition can readily be assessed with ultrasound without a need for a computed tomographic scan. Metabolic disturbances are often the basis for kidney stones in the pediatric population.

Advances in surgery are equally noteworthy, including closing gastroschisis, managing inguinal and other hernias, dealing with ovarian masses and torsion (emphasis on salvaging the ovary), and the surgical approach to pulmonary and pleural disorders, such as empyema, CPAM (congenital pulmonary airway malformations), and pneumothorax. Engagement in sports is on the rise with children being younger and often participating in a single sport with the subsequent development of overuse syndromes. In many cases, judicious pediatric advice and prevention are key to reducing such syndromes. Although once dismal, the prognosis for Duchenne muscular dystrophy is much improved with new developments related to the diagnosis, treatment, and management that have redefined the disease prognosis, course, and life expectancy.

As I write this Introduction, we are in the spring of 2020, amidst the COVID-19 pandemic. However, it's time to again plan for the 68th issue of *Advances in Pediatrics* and select subjects on which to report. Right now, it seems hard to believe there is interest in anything besides COVID-19, but there is. Fortunately, there continue to be new tools for diagnosis and new modalities for management. There will be new advances to report on as COVID-19 fades from the headlines.

Carol D. Berkowitz, MD, FAAP, FACEP
Division of General Pediatrics
Department of Pediatrics
Harbor-UCLA Medical Center
David Geffen School of Medicine at UCLA
1000 West Carson Street
Torrance, CA 90509, USA

E-mail address: cberkowitz52@gmail.com

Advances in Pediatrics 67 (2020) 1–13

ADVANCES IN PEDIATRICS

Collateral Damage

Mitigating Toxic Stress Secondary to Parental Military Service in Post-9/11 Military-Connected Children

Alicia Gill Rossiter, DNP*, Catherine J. Hernandez, MS, Konstance C. Mackie, MS

University of South Florida College of Nursing, 12901 Bruce B. Downs Boulevard, MDC 22, Tampa, Florida 33612, USA

Keywords

• Military-connected children • Military families • Post-9/11 • Military • Veteran • Toxic stress • Adverse childhood experiences • I serve 2

Key points

- Post-9/11 military-connected children (MCC) are at increased risk for physical, psychological, and behavioral health issues secondary to parental military service.
- Post-9/11 MCC are vulnerable to toxic stress secondary to deployments and relocations.
- Health care providers caring for post-9/11 MCC should be cognizant of their unique health care needs.
- Summary: health care providers who are knowledgeable with regard to military cultural competence identify post-9/11 MCC in their practices and incorporate the I Serve 2: A Pocketcard for Healthcare Providers Caring for Military Children, which could help mitigate the impact of toxic stress secondary to parental military service on post-9/11 MCC. Post-9/11 MCC are exposed to stressors not typically experienced by their civilian peers. Parental deployment and frequent relocation have a profound impact on developing children. Key to protecting this vulnerable population is appropriate screening and referral in the health care setting. Use of I Serve 2: A Pocketcard for Healthcare Providers Caring for Military Children at every encounter can aid with screening, guide providers in culturally competent care, and recommend appropriate resources and referrals in the community to mitigate the long-term effects of toxic stress on the physical, psychological, and behavioral wellness of MCC.

*Corresponding author. *E-mail address:* arossite@usf.edu
Twitter: @agr_drltc (A.G.R.)

https://doi.org/10.1016/j.yapd.2020.03.003

INTRODUCTION

Case report

Six-year-old Katie walks beside her father, Staff Sergeant (SSgt) Martinez. Skipping beside his wheelchair, she carries one of her father's prosthetic legs under her arm, and her father's other prosthetic leg lays across the arms of the wheelchair. SSgt Martinez was wounded in Afghanistan when his Humvee struck an improvised explosive device. In addition to having bilateral below-the-knee amputations, SSgt Martinez was also diagnosed with posttraumatic stress disorder (PTSD) and a traumatic brain injury (TBI) [1]. During his rehabilitation in the Washington, DC area, his family, including Katie, her 2 younger siblings, and her mother, moved from a military installation in the Midwest to the Washington, DC area to be closer to SSgt Martinez as he recovers from injuries and prepares to transition to civilian life after the injury. They have been living at the Fisher House for the past 5 weeks. Fisher Houses are scattered throughout the United States near military medical centers and Veterans' Affairs hospitals. The Fisher House Foundation is a nonprofit organization that provides a temporary home away from home for military family members to stay close to the medical centers where military members are being treated for illnesses and injuries sustained during deployments or other missions [2]. A nurse stops to speak to Katie and her father, who just finished a session with physical therapy, in which he is learning to walk with his new prosthetic limbs. Katie tells the nurse, "He's not my same daddy that went away to the war, but mommy said I need to be a big girl now and help take care of him. My daddy taught me how to walk when I was a little girl. Now I am going to be like my daddy and help him learn to walk." [1].

Military-connected children (MCC) make tremendous sacrifices in support of their parents' military service. An estimated 4 million children have a parent who is serving or has served in the military [3]. Resilient is the word most commonly used to describe military children, but 18 years of war is beginning to reveal the impact of parental military service on MCC and the stress/stressors these children face secondary to the military lifestyle, as well as the multiple deployments and/or relocations they experience. Although there is robust research focused on the impact of war on veterans and the physical and psychological stressors that war inflicts, less is known about the impact on MCC.

Critically important to ensuring the national security of the nation is ensuring that service members have the support and approval of their at-home spouses and the MCC; it is the leading factor determining whether or not service members continue to serve in the military [4]. Failure to achieve this leaves the United States with gaps in a fit fighting force and an economic burden when the average cost of training and retaining service members is considered [5]. Focusing on military families, to include military spouses and MCC, to meet their physical and psychological health, education, and employment needs is paramount to ensuring the success of not only the service members but also the military families [4]. This focus is more concerning in that less than 30% of eligible recruits across the nation between the ages of 18 and 24 years meet the physical and/or psychological requirements for military service because of obesity and comorbidities secondary to obesity (eg, diabetes and hypertension), deficits in education, other health issues, and incarceration, to name a few [6,7].

Furthermore, military service can be described as a family business. Approximately 80% of those who recently enlisted in the armed forces stated that they have at least 1 family member who had served, and more than 25% stated they had a parent who is serving or has served [8]. The inability to adequately support the physical, psychological, and behavioral health of MCC places their children at risk for health issues that may preclude them from future military service, should they choose to serve once they turn 18 years of age. In addition, the perception of a lack of consideration for military families may prevent MCC from continuing the lineage of family service in the military and place the nation at a deficit in meeting recruiting quotas, thereby affecting the security needs of the country.

Historically, the health care needs of MCC have gone unnoticed in the civilian population [9]. Lack of identification of MCC in clinics, hospitals, schools, and other health care settings places them at risk for stress and comorbidities associated with parental military service. More than 50% of active-duty MCC and 100% of Reserve, National Guard, and veteran children receive their health care in the civilian setting [10]. Therefore, it is critical that health care providers are educated and trained to identify MCC in civilian clinical practice and provide culturally competent care for this population to ensure the overall physical, psychological, and behavioral health of not only MCC but the entire military family.

Military-connected children: who are they?

Since the onset of the wars in Iraq and Afghanistan in 2001, military personnel have experienced more than 3.3 million deployments [11]. At present, there are approximately 1.3 million service members on active duty and another 815,000 serving in the Reserve and National Guard [12]. Roughly 39% of those who serve have family responsibilities (at least 1 child), including 38.4% of active duty personnel (n = 496,887) and 41.5% of Selected Reserve personnel (n = 338,257) [12]. More than 1.68 million children have the distinction of being called MCC [12]. These children are also young: 74% are 11 years of age or younger [12]. In addition, there are 2.1 million post-9/11 children of veterans [13]. Veterans are those who have separated from the military or retired and have assimilated back into civilian life. These MCC are a generation who have grown up knowing parental deployments and separations as the norm.

Blue Star children, those who have a parent serving in combat, have experienced multiple deployments over the past 18 years; some MCC have endured 10 or more deployments during their lifetimes. Many service members are returning to families with both the visible (polytrauma) and invisible (PTSD, TBI, and military sexual trauma) wounds of war, and the parents of service members, military spouses, and MCC are taking on caregiving responsibilities and an increased burden of care. There are 15,000 children classified as Gold Star children [14], which is the child of a service member who died while serving in combat.

The military culture and lifestyle provide many opportunities and experiences for MCC, and MCC live with a sense of patriotism and respect for the role their parents play in providing the safety and security of the nation, regardless of whether their parents are serving on active duty, in the Reserve or National Guard, or are veterans. However, research is starting to show the cumulative effect of 18 years of war that has exposed MCC to a large number of stressors and uncertainties, placing them at a higher risk for physical, psychological, and behavioral health issues and making them vulnerable to the effects of toxic stress. A recent report released by the Department of Defense, the first report on death by suicide in military family members, revealed that 186 military-connected family members (123 spouses and 63 dependents) committed suicide in calendar year 2017 [15]. Of note were the percentage of female spouses who committed suicide (69% of total spouse suicides), and the percentage of spousal suicides less than 40 years of age was 82% of total spouses. Furthermore, the report highlights that, of all dependents, spouses as well as children, more than 18 years of age (50% of total dependents) and dependents less than 18 years of age, particularly male dependents between the ages of 15 and 17 years, were at highest risk for suicide [15]. Therefore, there is a need for screening for depression and suicidal ideation not only in MCC but also in military spouses.

Research on stress and toxic stress is an emerging area focusing on the impact on the health and welfare of post-9/11 MCC and adolescents. Toxic stress occurs when the normal stress response (which can be a protective mechanism) is active but becomes extreme, frequent, or prolonged, leading to chronic health conditions such as depression, anxiety, autoimmune disease, certain cancers, and cardiovascular disease [16]. Although the research shows that military service is a risk factor for toxic stress in service members, less is known regarding the collateral damage (the unintended or incidental insults) post-9/11 MCC experience in support of their parents' military service.

Physiologic stress and the impact on physical health

MCC often experience the unintended or incidental health consequences of a parent's deployment. These issues stem from mental stress, which has the potential to alter the body's normal physiologic processes over time. The age and developmental level of each child should be taken into consideration, because stress can negatively affect brain growth and the attainment of developmental milestones [17,18].

Discovery of physiologic changes with stress

Hans Selye created the concept of the general adaptation syndrome in 1946 to describe the different stages of stress [19]. While observing rats during a laboratory experiment, he noted 3 distinct phases of adaptation to constant stress: (1) fight or flight; (2) physiologic compensation to altered homeostasis; and (3) a final stage, which is marked by the depletion of the subject's coping mechanisms and the body's loss of normal functioning, eventually leading to death [19]. More recently, the different types of responses to stress have been named based on the duration of the body's response. The shortest, most immediate stress response is called the positive stress response, because the body can quickly overcome its physiologic response to a stressor and return to a normal baseline. Preparation for an examination or going to a routine medical appointment are examples of causes of a positive stress response. Another stress response, called a tolerable stress response, happens when the body's alteration in homeostasis lasts for more than a few days to weeks. The body can still recover from potentially damaging physiologic responses, provided that the person who experiences tolerable stress has a good social support system or other positive coping skills. A divorce is an example of a cause of a tolerable stress response. Lastly, a toxic stress response is unrelieved stress on the body without social support or with maladaptive coping skills. This form of stress response can result from years of maltreatment or financial difficulties that cause a loss of food security. A toxic stress response eventually exhausts the body's self-healing capabilities. Chronic, debilitating health conditions ensue as a result of a toxic stress response [20]. No matter the cause of stress, the manner in which people appraise their own situations affects their overall well-being, both mentally and physically, and that translates from parents to their children [9,21,22].

How stress affects military-connected children

At-home parents whose spouses are deployed experience the same stressors as single parents by taking on the role of the absent parent and not having as many resources, such as time, to enable them to provide for the family or even to find respite care for themselves [17]. The psychological stress on a child's caregiver puts that child at a higher risk for maltreatment and neglect [10,17,23]. During deployment, there is an 11% decrease in well-child visits for MCC, but there is a corresponding 11% increase in visits for behavioral health issues. There are increases in visits to specialists and unplanned urgent care and emergency room visits as well [10,23,24]. Missed well-child examinations decrease the opportunities for providers to aid in identifying concerns before these problems escalate into acute or chronic phases of physical and mental illnesses.

In February 2020, the Defense Health Agency (DHA) announced some impactful changes to the Military Health System. One of these includes transitioning most active duty family member and retiree health care out of military treatment facilities to Tricare network civilian providers. Therefore, it is even more important for civilian providers to understand the health implications of the military lifestyle on military children, because a higher percentage of military children will no longer have access to health care from military providers [25].

How stress affects the body

Children who sense discord with the many changes that accompany the military lifestyle can experience negative health effects from the body's prolonged release of stress hormones. The release of these hormones in response to stress can have both positive and negative effects. A short burst of cortisol disbursed during temporary stress helps the body to more effectively provide glucose for energy and improves the distribution of protein to help heal any injured areas. In contrast, toxic stress causes stress hormones to potentiate each other, causing physical ailments such as peptic ulcers, hypertension, weight gain, and increased resting pulse [19].

Prolonged exposure to toxic stress, as seen with the dose-related effects of protracted and repeated deployments, not only increases anxiety and depression in MCC but also results in physical ramifications [24]. MCC may present with vague, somatic complaints, such as headaches and stomach aches [26,27]. One study determined that headaches increase in severity for 65% of military-connected girls aged 5 to 9 years during parental deployment. However, limited research has been done regarding somatic complaints in MCC. These symptoms are just as likely to be from depression or anxiety as they are from physiologic changes that the body undergoes with sustained stress [28]. For example, depression can masquerade as attention-deficit/hyperactivity disorder (ADHD), which may cause unnecessary or inappropriate medications to be prescribed. In younger, school-aged children who have difficulty verbally expressing emotions and self-regulating because of underlying depression, a teacher may erroneously suspect ADHD. This issue could be resolved by first ruling out stress and depression that could later manifest as physical ailments [9,26].

Parental stress increases a child's risk of maltreatment, with the most common form of maltreatment being neglect [10]. Neglect and prolonged stress can negatively affect brain growth [17,20]. During exposure to toxic stress, the brain prunes itself by phasing out specific neurons that are not stimulated and rewiring its pathways [20]. Milestones, such as verbal skills, may be delayed. With any pediatric health care visit, assessment of milestones can reveal problems early enough to provide appropriate interventions for the best outcomes [29,30]. As previously mentioned, well-child visits decrease during a parent's deployment. The increase in specialist visits may likely be from exacerbated problems that could have been ameliorated during a routine well-child visit, if caught earlier. However, barriers exist for MCC who need appropriate, specialized care. These barriers include parents assuming that their children will outgrow their problems, the sense that they can cope without professional assistance, lack of specialty providers, lack of providers who accept Tricare military insurance, and long waiting lists for appointments [29].

Behavioral and psychological impact

Navigating the continuous and often complex development in youth can be challenging, and research suggests that having a family member who is in the military and currently deployed, or has deployed with the military, further increases risks for dangerous decisions, disorders, and behaviors [10,18,24,31–38]. Bello-Utu and DeSocio [24] completed a systematic review of military child coping with both deployment and reintegration encompassing 27 publications. They found 3 predominant themes that influence child coping with parental deployment: (1) age and development of the child; (2) parental mental health, especially the at-home parent; and (3) previous resiliency influenced by length and number of deployments. Children's experience with parental deployments may expose them to extended periods of uncertainty and chronic toxic stress, diminishing their capability to cope [24,31,35,37]. Essentially, the impact of a parental deployment is thought to have a cumulative effect, or dose-response relationship, on the family unit. Therefore, longer or more numerous absences are reflected in poorer mental health for the deployed service member, at-home parent, and children left behind [10,31,32,39,40]. Furthermore, several studies identified discrepancies between parental perceptions of child behavior and coping, making their judgment of impending problems largely inaccurate [9,24,35,38]. In addition, service member parents with PTSD report considerable distress over parenting and are more likely to discipline severely [41]. Service members and their families who are reservists or members of the National Guard are at an even greater risk than their active duty counterparts of developing feelings of isolation, loneliness, and hopelessness, likely because these families typically reside in civilian communities, remote from military bases and military community support [10,24,31,35–38]. Although ability to cope is highly individualized, patterns of psychological/behavioral cues by age/development of the child have begun to emerge in the research.

Preschoolers

During parental deployment, younger children (birth to 5 years old) may show attachment concerns, sleep disturbances, increased comfort seeking, and separation anxiety, which may manifest as aggression or sadness [24]. Cramm and colleagues [32] noted that 12 studies focused on preschoolers, and most reported increased visits for mental health–related problems, behavioral concerns, and developmental delays related to deployment, noting separation anxiety, regression in toilet training, increase in incidences of crying, and oppositional behaviors.

School age

School-aged children (6–12 years old) most often reported worry, sadness, and anxiety during family member deployment, which may manifest as internalizing behaviors, such as declining academics, isolation, and withdrawal; or externalizing behaviors, such as increases in physical violence and anger. This behavior may result in an increased number of medical visits to emergency departments, urgent care, or specialty care [10,32].

Adolescents

Adolescents (11–19 years old) often showed similar behaviors to school-aged children; however, additional concerns present in the form of increased risk-taking behaviors, such as substance use, impulsive sexual activity, and suicidal thoughts and behaviors [24,32]. This age group has also shown increased victimization among their peers, gang involvement, weapon carrying, sadness, hopelessness, and disordered eating [24,31,34,42]. Also notable, a study by Tunac De Pedro and colleagues [38] found that older adolescents (>15 years of age) showed the greatest maladaptation to parental deployment of all age groups studied. For adolescents who may be struggling with navigating their own complex developments, it can become overwhelming, during parental deployment, to transition to a single-parent home and be expected to take on roles and responsibilities meant for an adult before being developmentally ready to do so [9,17,19,24,26].

A case for adverse childhood experiences in military children

In their groundbreaking study on adverse childhood experiences (ACEs), Felitti and colleagues [43] found that more than half of the 9508 respondents reported 1 or more exposures to abuse or family dysfunction in childhood. Furthermore, researchers associated these specific exposures in childhood with poorer physical and mental health in adulthood and linked them with several major causes of death in adults [43,44]. The researchers also concluded that parents who were subjected to ACEs were more likely to also expose their children to ACEs. In a small study of combat soldiers who sought treatment during deployment (n = 162), Applewhite and colleagues [45] found that 83% reported at least 1 ACE. This percentage is far higher than the 50% previously found by Felitti and colleagues [43] in their 1998 study of civilians exposed to ACEs. In addition, LeardMann and colleagues [46] studied the responses of 8391 male active duty Marines and found an increased risk for developing PTSD after returning from a deployment among respondents who also reported ACEs. Likewise, in their systematic review, Rodriguez and Margolin [47] discussed the profound effects of parental absence in childhood. That article compared temporary parental absence caused by military deployment, parental incarceration, or international migration and discovered similar themes among the 3 groups. The researchers recognized that, regardless of the rationale for the parental absence, the event is a significant stressor to the family unit and has broad, long-term consequences for the children.

Recommendations

- Use of the I Serve 2: A Pocketcard for Healthcare Providers Caring for Military Children initiative (Fig. 1) at every encounter helps health care providers identify and provide appropriate, definitive care for MCC, so that the effects of stress can be minimized for better health outcomes [9,10]. The pocketcard provides prompts for identification and assessment of military children, as well as referral and resources in the community. Historically, the use of pocketcards and clinical guidelines has been shown to improve health outcomes and quality

I SERVE 2: A POCKETCARD FOR HEALTHCARE PROVIDERS CARING FOR MILITARY CHILDREN©

I CARE Support Strategy for Military Children

- **Identify:**
  - Military children in your practice/community
  - Risk factors, mitigating aspects and patterns of coping
  - If the parent is Active Duty, Reservist, or National Guard in order to gauge services available
- **Correlate:**
  - Developmental stage, healthcare concerns in context of the individual child
  - Family and teacher concerns about child
- **Ask**
  - How the child is coping
  - Assess risks for physical, psychological, behavioral, social, and academic concerns
  - Conduct a vulnerability and safety assessment
  - How will the family ensure a smooth deployment and reintegration
  - What you can do to reduce unnecessary visits during deployment (e.g. medication refills, referrals, etc.)
- **Ready Resources**
  - Engage partnerships within the school system
  - Ready a list of local and national resources for military families
  - Encourage families to engage resources well in advance of deployment
  - Determine accessibility to military installation services
- **Encourage and educate**
  - Prevention strategies
  - Strong families and healthy problem solving
  - Early engagement with resources
  - Healthy expectations during and after deployment

I CARE created by Dr. Heather Johnson and Dr. Catherine G. Ling and adapted by Dr. Alicia Gill Rossiter DOI: 10.1111/1745-7599.12003

For additional information on I Serve 2 refer to: I Serve 2: Identifying and caring for militaryconnected children in civilian primary care settings—Dr. Alicia Gill Rossiter (arossite@usf.edu), Dr. Patricia A. Patrician, Dr. Mary Anne Dumas, Dr. Catherine Gaines Ling, Dr. Heather L. Johnson, and Dr. Margaret C. Wilmoth. DOI# 10.1097/JXX.0000000000000084. DOI: 10.1016/j.outlook.2016.05.01

Questions that can be asked of parents and military children at well child/acute care visits:

Correlate/Ask

•Has anyone expressed any concerns about you (or your child?)
•Have you noticed any of the following?

1. Increased stress
2. Anxiety, sadness
3. Emotional or physical outbursts
4. Crying/ overly emotional
5. Difficulty sleeping, nightmares
6. Difficulty concentrating
7. Change in academic performance or appetite
8. Clingy or distant
9. Increase in behavioral issues at home, school, with peers
10. Increase in complaints of stomach aches, headaches, or other physical symptoms

Ready Resources

•Who do you turn to for support? Where is this person located?
•What resources are available to you in the:

1. Military
2. Community
3. School/day care
4. Religious affiliations
5. Sports/ service organizations

Vulnerability/ risk assessments

•Where do you live? On or off a military instillation?
•Do you feel safe in your home?
•Are you concerned about your child?
•Tell me about the relationship with your parents.
•Tell me about a typical day at home/school
•How do you feel about your parent's job in the military?
•How have things been since your parent returned from deployment?

Copyright TXu 2-067-797 26 September 2017

I SERVE 2: A POCKETCARD FOR HEALTHCARE PROVIDERS CARING FOR MILITARY CHILDREN©

Military children make tremendous sacrifices in support of a parent(s) military service. Over 2 million children have a parent who is serving or has served in the Armed Forces. While "resilient" is the word used to describe most military children, it is important that we recognize the stresses/stressors of military life—that military children serve too—in order to support and care for them.

I SERVE 2

Ask your patients & their parents:

"Do you have a parent, sibling, or other family member who has ever served in the military?"

If the patient answers 'yes' ask:

- Is the military member:
  - Active duty?
  - Reservist?
  - National Guard?
  - Veteran?
- Has your parent deployed? Where? When?
- Where are you in the deployment cycle?
- What is your time for relocation (PCS)?

PREDEPLOYMENT (3 MONTHS BEFORE DEPARTURE): DENIAL, ANGER, SADNESS, FRUSTRATION
DEPLOYMENT (4 MONTHS TO 12 MONTHS): LONELINESS, FEAR, SLEEPLESSNESS, ANXIETY, ADJUSTING TO BEING ALONE, DETACHMENT, HIGH RISK FOR NEGLECT
REUNIFICATION (9 TO 12 MONTHS): APPREHENSION, ANTICIPATION, EXCITEMENT, EMOTIONAL READJUSTMENT, HIGH RISK FOR ABUSE

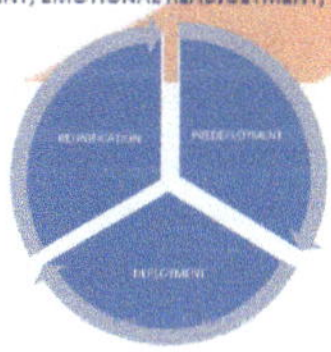

RESOURCES

BLUE STAR FAMILIES: WWW.BLUESTARFAM.ORG/RESOURCES/DEPLOYMENTS/DEPLOYMENT-RESOURCES/

CHILD MIND INSTITUTE: WWW.CHILDMIND.ORG/TOPICS/CONCERNS/MILITARY-FAMILIES/

MILITARY.COM: HTTP://WWW.MILITARY.COM/SPOUSE/MILITARY-LIFE/MILITARY-RESOURCES/FAMILY-SUPPORT-SERVICES.HTML

MILITARY ONE SOURCE: WWW.MILITARYONESOURCE.MIL

MILITARY CHILD EDUCATION COALITION: WWW.MILITARYCHILD.ORG

NATIONAL MILITARY FAMILY ASSOCIATION: WWW.MILITARYFAMILY.ORG

U.S DEPARTMENT OF EDUCATION: WWW.ED.GOV/VETERANS-AND-MILITARY-FAMILIES

Fig. 1. I Serve 2: A Pocketcard for Healthcare Providers Caring for Military Children. (*Courtesy of* Alicia Gill Rossiter, DNP, Tampa, FL.)

of care when integrated into clinical practice [48]. The American Academy of Nursing and Veterans' Affairs have developed pocketcards for use by health care providers caring for veterans in the civilian sector and these were used as exemplars in the development of the I Serve 2: A Pocketcard for Healthcare Providers Caring for Military Children.

- The ICARE (identify, correlate, ask, ready resources, and encourage/educate) support strategy delineated in the I Serve 2: A Pocketcard for Healthcare Providers Caring for Military Children gives health care providers a strategy designed to build resilience and develop healthy problem solving critical to the mission of building healthy military families, while mitigating the impact of toxic stress secondary to parental military service on MCC.
- Critical to the success of working with military families is decreasing the stigma of seeking professional help by discussing this as an enhancement to care with military families. This approach will help to promote acceptance of the importance of mental health care.
- Health care provider referral of military families to available resources, such as the Family Advocacy Program, can assist to proactively strengthen communication within the family or work with the Department of Child and Family Services to more effectively monitor highly transient military families who may have a history of discord [10].
- Unique identifiers added to electronic medical records act as cognitive reminders for providers to ask the necessary questions of military families to optimize their care [18].
- Promoting continuing education by professional organizations and licensure bodies for physicians, advanced practice registered nurses, physician assistants, and registered nurses about the needs of military families will reduce the current knowledge gap of providers and can be used as a condition of continuing licensure [9]. In addition, inclusion of veteran health competencies in health care–related programs, such as the ones listed earlier, would provide baseline knowledge and education.
- Parents are often concerned about their children's milestones. With current technology, parents have applications at their fingertips that can help them monitor their children's growth and development. This technology may encourage parents to bring their children in for well-child examinations, especially if a parent suspects a problem. One such application is the Centers for Disease Control and Prevention's Milestone Tracker app, which can be downloaded onto a smartphone [30].
- Increasing access to military and community-based resources for military parents will encourage their use. Emotionally available parents who have positive coping mechanisms can help to mitigate the negative health effects of stress on their children [21,29].
- Securing research funding by engaging stakeholders for the purpose of increasing the body of evidence regarding the impact of military service on families and how to best meet the unique health care needs of military families.

SUMMARY

Post-9/11 MCC are exposed to stressors not typically experienced by their civilian peers. Parental deployment and frequent relocation have a profound impact on developing children. Key to protecting this vulnerable population is appropriate screening and referral in the health care setting. Use of I Serve 2: A Pocketcard for Healthcare Providers Caring for Military Children at every encounter can guide providers in the delivery of culturally competent care and provide recommendations for appropriate resources and referrals in the community that can mitigate the long-term effects of toxic stress on the physical, psychological, and behavioral wellness of MCC.

Disclosure

The views expressed in this article reflect the results of research conducted by the authors and do not necessarily reflect the official policy or position of the University of South Florida, Department of the Navy or Air Force, Department of Defense, nor the United States Government.

I am a military service member or federal/contracted employee of the United States government. This work was prepared as part of my official duties. Title 17 U.S.C. 105 provides that 'copyright protection under this title is not available for any work of the United States Government.' Title 17 U.S.C. 101 defines a U.S. Government work as work prepared by a military service member or employee of the U.S. Government as part of that person's official duties.

References

[1] Biden Foundation. I Serve 2: Identifying and caring for military-connected kids in a clinical setting. Available at: https://archive.bidenfoundation.org/news/i-serve-2-identifying-and-caring-for-military-connected-kids-in-a-clinical-setting/. Accessed October 15, 2019.

[2] Fisher House. Available at: https://fisherhouse.org/. Accessed February 27, 2020.

[3] Nelson SC, Baker MJ, Weston CG. Impact of military deployment on the development and behavior of children. Pediatr Clin North Am 2016;63(5):795–811.

[4] Meadows SO, Tanielian T, Karney B, et al. The deployment life study: longitudinal analysis of military families across the deployment cycle. Rand Health Q 2016;6(2):7. Available at: https://www.rand.org/pubs/periodicals/health-quarterly/issues/v6/n2/07.html. Accessed October 15, 2019.

[5] Dahlman R. The cost of a military person-year. A method for computing savings from force reductions. Washington, DC: Rand National Defense Research Institute; 2007. Available at: https://www.rand.org/content/dam/rand/pubs/monographs/2007/RAND_MG598.pdf. Accessed October 21, 2019.

[6] Mission Readiness. Too fat to fight: Retired military leaders want junk food out of America's schools. Mission Readiness: Military leaders for Kids 2010. Available at: http://cdn.missionreadiness.org/MR_Too_Fat_to_Fight-1.pdf. Accessed October 30, 2019.

[7] Centers for Disease Control and Prevention. Unfit to serve: Obesity is impacting national security. 2019. Available at: https://www.cdc.gov/physicalactivity/downloads/unfit-to-serve.pdf. Accessed October 30, 2019.

[8] Thompson M. Here's why the U. S. military is a family business. Time Magazine 2016. Available at: https://time.com/4254696/military-family-business/. Accessed October 30, 2019.

[9] Rossiter AG, Patrician PA, Dumas MA, et al. I Serve 2: Identifying and caring for military-connected children in civilian primary care settings. J Am Acad Nurse Pract 2018;30(11):614–20.

[10] Huebner CR. Health and mental health needs of children in US military families. Pediatrics 2019;143(1):1–13.

[11] Sheppard SC, Malatras JW, Israel AC. The impact of deployment on U.S. military families. Am Psychol 2010;65(6):599–609.
[12] Department of Defense. Demographics: Profile of the military community. 2017. Available at: https://download.militaryonesource.mil/12038/MOS/Reports/2017-demographics-report.pdf. Accessed October 30, 2019.
[13] Hanson D, Woods T. The state of post 9/11 veteran families. Available at: https://www.urban.org/sites/default/files/publication/85986/the_state_of_post-911_veteran_families_final_last_11_21_2016.pdf. Accessed November 15, 2019.
[14] Taylor V. Gold star children act. Available at: https://vantaylor.house.gov/uploadedfiles/van_taylor_gold_star_children_summary.pdf. Accessed October 15, 2019.
[15] Department of Defense. Annual suicide report. 2018. Available at: https://assets.documentcloud.org/documents/6432219/2018-DoD-Annual-Suicide-Report-FINAL-25-SEP-19.pdf. Accessed October 30, 2019.
[16] Johnson SB, Riley AW, Granger DA, et al. The science of early life toxic stress for pediatric practice and advocacy. Pediatrics 2013;131(2):319–27.
[17] Boberiene LV, Hornback BJ. How can policy strengthen community support for children in military families? Am J Orthopsychiatry 2014;84(5):439–46.
[18] Panton J. Caring for military children: Implications for nurse practitioners. J Pediatr Health Care 2018;32(5):435–44.
[19] McCance KL, Huether SE. Stress and disease. In: Brashers VL, Rote NS, editors. Pathophysiology: the biologic basis for disease in adults and children. St Louis (MO): Elsevier Mosby; 2014. p. 338–62.
[20] Center on the Developing Child: Harvard University. Toxic stress. Available at: https://developingchild.harvard.edu/science/key-concepts/toxic-stress/?fbclid=IwAR2tnmWmQOckHxZ76F_Rs3aYHXJ42XVoROqZLQf3JSMEy74GhSjaMNZF2I. Accessed November 7, 2019.
[21] Cederbaum JA, Gilreath TD, Benbenishty R, et al. Well-being and suicidal ideation of secondary school students from military families. J Adolesc Health Care 2014;54(6):672–7.
[22] Gewirtz AH, DeGarmo DS, Zamir O. After deployment, adaptive parenting tools: 1-year outcomes of an evidence-based parenting program for military families following deployment. Prev Sci 2018;19(4):589–99.
[23] Trautmann J, Alhusen J, Gross D. Impact of deployment on military families with young children: A systematic review. Nurs Outlook 2015;63(6):656–79.
[24] Bello-Utu CF, DeSocio JE. Military deployment and reintegration: A systematic review of child coping. J Child Adolesc Psychiatr Nurs 2015;28(1):23–34.
[25] Military Health System. Restructuring and realignment of military medical treatment facilities. Available at: https://health.mil/About-MHS/OASDHA/Defense-Health-Agency/Congressional-Relations/Restructuring-and-Realignment-of-Military-Medical-Treatment-Facilities. Accessed March 1, 2020.
[26] Hamilton L, Ling C, Rossiter AG. Impact of parental military service on the health of military-connected children: A case study. J Pediatr Health Care 2018;32(6):634–8.
[27] Hathaway A, Russotti J, Metzger J, et al. Meeting military children's biopsychosocial needs: Exploring evidence-based interventions. Best Pract Ment Health 2018;14(1, Pt 2):54–77. Available at: http://search.ebscohost.com.ezproxy.hsc.usf.edu/login.aspx?direct=true&db=psyh&AN=2018-08775-006&site=ehost-live. Accessed October 16, 2019.
[28] Swedean SK, Gonzales MV, Zickefoose BA, et al. Recurrent headache in military-dependent children and the impact of parent deployment. Mil Med 2013;178(3):274–8.
[29] Flittner O'Grady AE, MacDermid Wadsworth S, Willerton E, et al. Help seeking by parents in military families on behalf of their young children. Psychol Serv 2015;12(3):231–40.
[30] Centers for Disease Control. CDC's milestone tracker app. Available at: https://www.cdc.gov/ncbddd/actearly/milestones-app.html. Accessed November 8, 2019.
[31] Alfano CA, Lau S, Balderas J, et al. The impact of military deployment on children: Placing developmental risk in context. Clin Psychol Rev 2016;43:17–29.

[32] Cramm H, McColl MA, Aiken AB, et al. The mental health of military-connected children: A scoping review. J Child Fam Stud 2019;28:1725–35.
[33] Estrada JN, Gilreath TD, Sanchez CY, et al. Associations between school violence, military connection, & gang membership in California secondary schools. Am J Orthopsychiatry 2017;87:443–51.
[34] Gilreath TD, Wrabel SL, Sullivan KS, et al. Suicidality among military-connected adolescents in California schools. Suicidality among military-connected adolescents in California schools. Eur Child Adolesc Psychiatry 2016;25:61–6.
[35] Johnson HL, Ling CG. Caring for military children in the 21st century. J Am Acad Nurse Pract 2013;25:195–202.
[36] Kelly D, Paul M. Veterans-by-proxy: A conceptual framework of ambiguous loss among children of combat veterans. J Fam Soc Work 2018;21(4–5):255–70.
[37] Ling CG, Johnson HL. Caring for military children in the emergency department: The essentials. J Emerg Nurs 2013;39(6):648–51.
[38] Tunac De Pedro K, Astor RA, Gilreath TD, et al. School climate, deployment, and mental health among students in military-connected schools. Youth Soc 2018;50(1):93–115.
[39] Creech SK, Hadley W, Borsari B. The impact of military deployment and reintegration on children and parenting: A systematic review. Prof Psychol Res Pr 2014;45(6):452–64.
[40] Kuehner CA. My military: A navy nurse practitioner's perspective on military culture and joining forces for veteran health. J Am Acad Nurse Pract 2013;25:7–83.
[41] Chesmore AA, He Y, Zhang N, et al. Parent discrepancies in ratings of child behaviors following wartime deployment. J Trauma Stress 2018;31:79–88.
[42] Schvey NA, Sbrocco T, Stephens M, et al. Comparison of overweight and obese military-dependent and civilian adolescent girls with loss-of-control eating. Int J Eat Disord 2015;48(6):790–4.
[43] Felitti VJ, Anda RF, Nordenberg D, et al. Relationship of childhood abuse and household dysfunction to many of the leading causes of death in adults: the adverse childhood experiences (ACE) study. Am J Prev Med 1998;14(4):245–58.
[44] Arincorayan D, Applewhite L, Garrido M, et al. Resilience-enhancing relationships: What we can learn from those with a history of adverse childhood experiences. US Army Med Dep J 2017;2(17):25–32.
[45] Applewhite L, Arincorayan D, Adams B. Exploring the prevalence of adverse childhood experiences in soldiers seeking behavioral health care during a combat deployment. Mil Med 2016;181(10):1275–80.
[46] LeardMann CA, Smith B, Ryan MAK. Do adverse childhood experiences increase the risk of post deployment posttraumatic stress disorder in US Marines? BMC Public Health 2010;10:4. Available at: https://bmcpublichealth.biomedcentral.com/articles/10.1186/1471-2458-10-437. Accessed November 05, 2019.
[47] Rodriguez AJ, Margolin G. Parental incarceration, transnational migration, and military deployment: Family process mechanisms of youth adjustment to temporary parent absence. Clin Child Fam Psychol Rev 2015;18:24–49.
[48] BootsMiller BJ, Yankey JW, Flach SD, et al. Classifying the effectiveness of Veterans Affairs guideline implementation effectiveness. Am J Med Qual 2004;19:248–54.

Advances in Pediatrics 67 (2020) 15–28
ADVANCES IN PEDIATRICS

Using the Attachment Relationship and Positive Parenting Principles to Build Childhood Resilience

Sasha Svendsen, MD[a,*], Jessica Griffin, PsyD[b], Heather Forkey, MD[a]

[a]Child Protection Program and Foster Children Evaluation Services (FaCES), Department of Pediatrics, UMass Memorial Children's Medical Center, University of Massachusetts Medical School, 55 Lake Avenue North, Worcester, MA 01655, USA; [b]Child Trauma Training Center, Department of Psychiatry, University of Massachusetts Medical School, 55 Lake Avenue North, Worcester, MA 01655, USA

Keywords

• Attachment • Resilience • Positive parenting

Key points

- Attachment is the foundation for building childhood resilience.
- The security that comes from attachment relationships is the best way to support growth and development and regulate emotional distress.
- The attributes of resilience are best developed and supported by positive parenting techniques.
- Using positive parenting principles can support and reinforce the attachment relationship.

INTRODUCTION

As the impact of adversity and trauma on child development, behavior and lifelong health has been elucidated, there have been calls for the promotion of resilience in the pediatric setting [1,2]. Yet, *how* this can be accomplished in the pediatric medical setting has not been as clearly described. It turns out that pediatric medical

*Corresponding author. *E-mail address:* Sasha.Svendsen@umassmemorial.org

https://doi.org/10.1016/j.yapd.2020.04.004
0065-3101/20/

providers are well-positioned to do just this through their role supporting attachment relationships and developing caregiver skills within the clinical setting.

Resilience, defined by Masten, is a dynamic process of positive adaptation to or despite significant adversities [3]. Others have identified resilience as the ability not just to bounce back, but to "bounce forward" [4]. Masten further explains that this is achieved through the give and take of safe, stable, nurturing relationships that are continuous over time (attachment), and in the developmental growth, that occurs through play, exploration and exposure to a variety of routine activities and resources (building skills) [3].

Pediatric medical providers attend to attachment in every patient encounter by observing and responding based on the reported and observed caregiver and child dynamic. And yet, many consider the topic of attachment to be challenging, confusing, and some of the methodology used to address attachment in prior decades to be concerning. It is often not a formal part of pediatric medical education and training. Although attachment disorders have been described in the literature since the 1950s, there was little research or exploration of the topic until the mid 1990s. Pediatric medical providers are often confused by the terminology, scope, evolution, and significance of attachment and attachment disorders within the clinical setting [5]. That need not be the case. By gaining some comfort with the fundamental features of attachment and simple ways to foster it through positive parenting practices, pediatric medical providers have a unique opportunity to promote resilience skills in children and their caregivers.

WHAT DO WE NEED TO KNOW ABOUT RESILIENCE?

If resilience is defined as a *dynamic* process of positive adaptation to or despite significant adversities, then it is not a fixed competency or characteristic, but includes skills that can be modeled, taught, practiced, reinforced, and learned. Resilience is often misunderstood to be a characteristic you either have or do not have. It is not a static process, but rather a set of competencies that can be grown and developed. Masten provided a list of these adaptive mechanisms that lead to resilience, a list that can be reorganized to form a mnemonic, THREADS [3].

The THREADS or resilience factors are:

- *T*hinking and learning brain (with opportunity for continued growth; cognitive development)
- *H*ope (optimism, faith and belief in a future for one's self)
- *R*egulation or self-control
- *E*fficacy (knowing one can impact one's environment and situation)
- *A*ttachment (having a secure attachment)
- *D*evelopmental skill mastery (of age-salient developmental tasks)
- *S*ocial connectedness (the larger network of relationships in which one lives and learns)

We are not born with these skills and need to learn and develop them over time. In fact, they represent significant developmental milestones to be achieved throughout childhood and are an important component of anticipatory guidance provided to caregivers within the clinical setting.

The development of the human brain begins before birth and continues throughout the lifespan. However, this brain development is especially rapid during the first 3 years of life, based on genetics and early life experience. For children, those experiences are primarily within the context of the caregiving relationship. One of the key principles in neurodevelopment is the brain's capacity to organize and develop in a use-dependent fashion. The more the brain is activated through positive, repetitive "serve and return" [6,7] interactions with caregivers, the stronger those brain connections become. Skills children learn and cultivate through these interactions (eg, self-regulation, awareness, planning, and flexibility) become the foundation for their physical and mental health, behavior and interactions in the world, and their future resilience [8]. Thus, it is relationships that are the fundamental adaptational mechanisms upon which resilience skills build, with the attachment relationship between the child and their caregiver being the most critical.

Attachment is the essential baseline skill for building resilience. Although it is helpful to remember the resilience factors, the THREADS mnemonic does not prioritize the attributes of resilience. Yet attachment is the primary one. It is critical to recognize that all the other adaptational skills develop in the context of attachment to a competent caregiver and the supports that the attachment relationship provides. This is not just limited to early childhood and, in fact, occurs throughout the lifespan; as children age into adulthood, other types of attachment relationships (eg, romantic attachment) can continue to foster resilience [9].

THE CHARACTERISTICS OF ATTACHMENT

Affectional bonds all involve a desire for closeness, distress with separation, joy with reunification, and grief upon loss of the cherished person. But attachment to a competent caregiver is distinct, in that the competent caregiver provides security and comfort to the child in the face of distress [10]. The image that many think of when they hear the word "attachment" is that of a caregiver holding or soothing an infant. When an infant is distressed, the infant looks to the caregiver. Infants are not born attached to the caregiver, but are born "hardwired" to seek the safety and support of specific caregivers. From an evolutionary standpoint, this process promotes children staying close to the adults who can protect them from predators. As children achieve this proximity, the communication developed between the caregiver and child begins the process of a child learning to interact with others, understand themselves, and regulate their own emotions [5].

The attachment relationship of child to caregiver begins at birth as the infant makes eye contact, hears the voices, and is fed and held by an attentive caregiver. In healthy relationships, the caregiver responds by providing empathy appropriate to the distress and needs of the child. Another way of explaining what the caregiver does is "attunement," which most literally means "bringing into harmony" [11]. Even when the child is not distressed, the caregiver is "in tune" with the child, providing support that matches the child's needs in tempo, rhythm, and volume. Mental health literature often refers to this as "psychological holding," an image that mirrors the physical act of cradling, protecting, and providing security [10,12].

That caregiver then forms the "secure base" from which children can explore and a "safe haven" to return to when there is threat or danger [13]. This process not only helps to calm the child's stress response, but also allows for emotional regulation to be restored during times of distress [14]. A child's ability to explore and learn through interaction with their physical and social environments as they gain motor skills is linked to the presence and functioning of this secure base and safe haven. Over time, the child learns to expect this response from the caregiver, to trust that the caregiver is predictable and will take care of the child's needs.

When a child is confident that the caregiver will be predictably and compassionately available, they are empowered to explore, learn, and gain other developmental skills. Reflected in and demonstrated by this consistent caregiver, children develop early and consistent working maps of themselves and the world, and learn how social relationships work. Ironically, dependence (eg, on a caregiver) fosters independence in the child. In contrast, if the child experiences fear or distress in the physical or social environment, this exploration and development is abandoned as the child seeks the safety of the caregiver [5,15]. Thus, attachment, this affiliative relationship that provides safety, becomes the lynchpin for how a child interacts with the world, understands himself or herself, experiences relationships with others, and develops skills in regulating his or her own emotions.

THE BUILDING BLOCKS OF ATTACHMENT

Although children are hardwired to attach, attachment does not just happen. It is the result of some very specific emotional supports that a caregiver provides to a child in the context of their relationship. These include:

- Safety and security
- Predictable compassionate availability
- Emotional container
- Attunement or "mentalizing" [16] (keeping the mind in mind)

The concept of safety and security is the fundamental feature of attachment. If separated from a caregiver, the child's cries of distress alert the caregiver to the child's need for protection. Attachment, that safe space for the child, also provides them with a secure base for exploration. Take the example of a toddler on a playground–the child moves away from the caregiver as they investigate the equipment, checks back with their caregiver to get more support, and then returns to play. Like an accordion, secure attachment fluctuates between closeness and distance while always remaining connected. The safe haven and the secure base that attachment creates for children ultimately provide them with a sense of psychological security so they are able to go out and explore their environment. It is through this security in attachment and security in exploration that children not only develop confidence in others, but also in the world around them, and perhaps most importantly, confidence in themselves.

Predictable compassionate availability is that measured, consistent response, reliably provided to the child by the caregiver [17]. When the child is distressed or dysregulated, the primary caregiver comforts the child through psychological attunement to the child's distress. By anticipating empathy from their caregiver, the child is confident in turning to this caregiver for comfort in times of distress.

Children need the caregiver to tolerate distress and emotion, thus allowing the child to recognize what the emotion is and name it. Only when the child is able to first identify an emotion can the child then develop the ability to modulate that emotion. In so doing, caregivers provide an emotional container for the child, recognizing that the child may have strong emotions, and although the emotion is expressed with the caregiver, it is not usually about the caregiver [18]. To do this, caregivers must have control and mastery over their own emotions. The dysregulated adult finds it difficult to provide this skill for a dysregulated child. Caregivers need to learn to tolerate those emotions from the child, because it is the emotions that are going to allow the child to learn to self-regulate–and unless any and all emotions can be tolerated–the child will not learn to identify, express, modulate, and manage those feelings (eg, the skills of regulation).

Finally, caregivers must look at the world through the child's eyes, or to keep the child's mind in mind. This concept from the mental health literature is also referred to as "mentalizing." [19] This skill is required not just for attachment, but for all the THREADS. Like learning to speak by being spoken to, we learn to understand our emotions by having responsive caregivers reflect and be attuned to our emotions. Consider the example of the infant crying owing to hunger. A caregiver picks up the child and says, "There, there. You're hungry, and we're going to get you a bottle right now." The child learns in these interactions what the distressing feeling is, and that the caregiver will help them to manage and resolve their distress. Alternatively, the reprimanding response a child receives from a caregiver of, "Shut up, you stupid kid. Are you just trying to bother me?" may be the result of the caregiver's own mental health issues, substance use, or other stressors. That child internalizes a very different understanding of self and the world–the feeling they have is of being stupid, not hungry, that the caregiver cannot help them to address the issue of need, and, in fact, there is no support available. For that child, their own feelings and needs are dangerous or represent failings, and the world is perceived as dangerous and unsupportive.

Although used interchangeably at times, bonding and attachment are not the same. Children attach to their caregivers, whereas caregivers bond to their children. Children are not expected to provide predictable compassionate availability, safety, emotional containment, or to look at the world through the caregiver's perspective. When caregivers expect this of children, the relationship is not healthy and these are children who grow up in "parentified" roles, leading to a number of negative outcomes for these youth [20].

Medical providers model all of these supports for caregivers. Patients and families can attach to consistent medical providers, and medical providers develop bonded relationships with the families served. In this way, the components of attachment can be demonstrated and taught to caregivers. By holding the emotions of caregivers who are frightened, frustrated, or confused, pediatric medical providers provide safety and predictable compassionate availability. Day after day, the work of the pediatric medical provider is to see the world from the patient and family's eyes.

In summary, this is empathy–the ability to see the world as another sees it, and to see another person as they see themselves, apart from external perceptions. It is the sum of the caregiver providing safety, predictable compassionate availability, being an emotional container and doing so with the child's mind in mind. Empathy implies a positive regard, which requires acceptance, affirmation, caring, nonpossessive warmth, and the valuing of another person as a unique individual. It is characterized by congruence, genuineness and authenticity [10].

This is what pediatric medical providers do within every patient encounter, whether we realize it or not. It is in these moments that pediatric medical providers expand their role within the clinical encounter to support the attachment of children to caregivers, by first providing empathy to the caregiver. It involves putting aside constrained professionalism and behaving more naturally [10]. Attuned, attentive listening is one way we project empathy to the caregiver or child, by making them feel "heard." Caregivers cannot give to their children what they themselves do not have. Empathy provided by the pediatric medical provider helps to decrease caregiver and child distress and opens the space for the caregiver to empathize with the child and models how they can do so.

A PROPOSED CONCEPTUAL FRAMEWORK

With a solid base of attachment, children can continue the process of developing resilience through the other adaptive mechanisms. None of these are learned and mastered, but each develops and grows over time, building step by step. Most of the time, children grow in all of these skills almost spontaneously. Through the give and take of safe stable nurturing relationships, these skills evolve naturally, advancing a child's ability to manage increasingly complex ideas about themselves, others, the world and how to negotiate within it. This is why Masten calls the process "ordinary magic" [3].

The strings behind the magic trick are the "THREADS." It is only when the magic does not happen that we realize key steps are missing. This is why evidence-informed therapies and evidence-based treatment that support children who have experienced trauma are organized to rebuild these capacities in a staged or stepwise fashion [21,22]. Similarly, we can reorganize the

THREADS into a stepwise process. To manage a level up, the capacity below it must be firmly established.

This staircase model provides a conceptual framework for the process by which we are most resilient (Fig. 1). In fact, all humans go up and down the steps each day, and all are their most resilient when these steps are supported and promoted. The more consistent the support, the more these competencies are strengthened. Attachment is the first step. It supports regulation and self-control. Regulation in turn, allows for the use of the thinking and learning brain and developmental skill mastery. With regulation, one then has the physiologic, cognitive, and emotional organization to further develop skills and to learn. This regulation, learning, and skill mastery results in a sense of efficacy. Self-efficacy then allows one to see a future for oneself where success is possible. With that perspective, one can think about a future resulting in hope. Social connectedness is the railing along this "staircase," supporting the child all the way up the stairs.

Looking at each of these steps a little more closely, there are some practical strategies that pediatric medical providers can recommend to caregivers that can help to support each of the resilience attributes along the way. These strategies include various positive parenting techniques and can be applied across the various ages and stages of childhood and adolescent development.

Attachment

Attachment is fundamental. As noted elsewhere in this article, demonstrating empathy and modeling the safety, predictable compassionate availability,

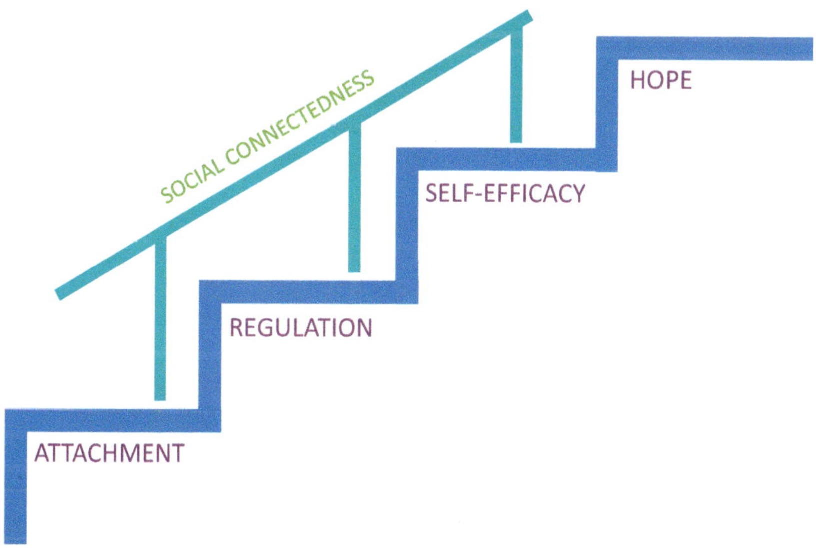

Fig. 1. Conceptual framework for the attributes of resilience.

emotional container, and keeping the mind in mind are all ways pediatric medical providers start to support attachment relationships.

To support strong and healthy attachment, these are some tools to consider.

Quality time in

Quality time is a fundamental aspect of caregiving that is, a common, recommended everyday practice. Although it may look a bit different at each age and developmental stage, the key to this principle is the caregiver spending time with the infant, child, or teen in a way in which the caregiver is truly present. During this time, the caregiver is fully focused and engaged with the child and distractions are minimized. "Serve and return" begins in the newborn period and continues throughout childhood, which evolves into attuned, attentive listening and conversation as a child matures.

Special time

The special time technique is a more specific form of quality time in that can help to reawaken empathy and attachment in situations where it is strained [23]. First, the frustrated caregiver and child are provided with the opportunity to express those relationship strains to the medical provider, who listens with empathy, validating the emotion and strain. Then they are given "homework" to carve out a child-directed activity (which cannot be chores and must be an activity the child chooses, at a time the parent chooses, so they can both be fully present and engaged). Once at home, at the appointed time, for 15 minutes the parent is to follow the child's lead and participate in whatever activity the child has chosen. The caregiver must focus on the child and the activity, with no other distractions. There should be a well-defined end to the time.

This time needs to be followed up with another meeting with the pediatric medical provider to discuss and review. Sometimes, behavior will worsen toward the end of the activity, or just after it has completed–indicating that this technique is ... working! Having had "special time" with a caregiver's attuned attention, the child does not want to lose it, and the increased protests of a child may be their attempt to return to that attuned relationship. In follow-up, the caregivers should be supported to repeat and expand elements of the interaction in other settings, increasing the caregiver's empathy for and attunement to the child. Over time, with this renewed connection, the child's behavior will usually improve and attachment will be strengthened.

These techniques do not end in childhood and can be practiced well into adolescence. For example, special time can be practiced with a caregiver and a teenager, by having the teenager show the caregiver how to use an app on their phone or learn a dance move, cook a meal together, and so on.

Attuned, attentive, and empathic listening

Attuned, attentive, and empathic listening is a consistent "serve and return" over time and part of "quality time in," yet deserves particular attention because it is affirming and creates a safe space for a child to explore ideas. By providing attuned, attentive, empathic listening, the caregiver effectively acts as an emotional container for the child. It models and reinforces healthy relationship skills. When the caregiver engages the child in problem solving while positively reflecting back to the child, it models self-regulation and is experienced by the child as predicable compassionate availability.

Regulation

Regulation is the act of managing one's thoughts and feelings to engage in goal-directed behaviors. Regulation is a foundational skill for future development, and one that has emotional, cognitive, and behavioral components [24,25]. Regulation is the result of first identifying emotions and then modulating them. It is the development of these skills over time that creates the scaffolding on which more advanced skills emerge and build on themselves. During childhood, self-regulation is the ability to calm oneself, delay gratification, or modulate responses for brief periods of time. During adolescence, self-regulation develops to include things like the ability to organize time and responsibilities, use increasingly complex cognitive strategies to manage internal distress, and problem solve while in emotionally charged situations [24]. This process also occurs in a step-wise fashion. The caregiver must be regulated themselves, then dyadically coregulate the child, using attuned responses to actively influence a child's experience. By the caregiver reflecting, mirroring, and modeling behavior, the child gradually internalizes these skills, thus developing self-regulation.

The parenting activities that can best support the development of a child's self-regulation include routines and rituals, Rewards and privileges, time out, and ignoring or distracting from minor negative behavior.

Routines and rituals

Routines and rituals are some of the most effective ways to help children develop a sense of safety and security. Having a predictable and consistent routine allows children to know what to expect and count on; they learn to self-regulate when they can predict and prepare for what is coming next. Predictable routines that promote self-regulation allow children to learn to control their impulses and increase their tolerance for frustrations, and begin to develop a sense of accomplishment and mastery [26]. When possible, giving the child some choices in the routine can also be very helpful, because it fosters a sense of control.

Children thrive on predictable but flexible routines. Some daily routines in today's modern world are outside of our control and are structured around work schedules, childcare, school, and other activities, rather than on the child's innate rhythms. Although this circumstance can be challenging, there are ways to address it. One way to take back routine and rhythm is to schedule the important things first. Some great examples of this are set family meal times and regular family nights, both of which are examples of ways to dedicate some "time in" with the people we love and value the most.

Rewards and privileges

Working for a reward is not just a childish pursuit. Adults earn paychecks and are financially rewarded for hard work. These positive demonstrations of achievement are not bribes, but rather a means of rewarding the building of skills. Some examples might include:

- A small amount of screen time in the evening for a child who has completed homework and handed it in on time
- A child completing a chore chart to earn a sleep-over

The reward must be desirable to the child and it is helpful if the child can have some say in choosing the rewards. At least initially, the reward should be small and easy to earn so it becomes reinforcing. This process develops executive functioning areas of the brain as the child has to wait, organize, and complete tasks. Reward systems are widely used in parenting and behavioral management programs with challenging youth–because they work. However, it is important that rewards and privileges not be the only skill a caregiver uses.

Time out

Many caregivers use time out as their first go to. For a time out to be most effective, it should be used judiciously. This strategy is only useful once attachment is established and secure, and is used more as a tool to promote regulation. It requires that there has been sufficient quality time in and special time, otherwise it has no value. Threatening a time out as a punishment is a misuse of the tool. The purpose of a time out is to prevent a behavior from escalating and to increase the child's ability to self-soothe and/or modulate their behavior and affect. Sometimes, the phrase "time out" has a pejorative context and just renaming "time out" to "taking space" or going to the child's "cozy corner" can help to make this technique more effective. In general, the time out should last 1 minute per year of age, be held in a neutral location (no distractions, television, etc.) and within eyesight of a caregiver. Caregivers can use a kitchen timer and, as soon as the time out is over, resume normal activities, looking for an opportunity to catch the child being good (described elsewhere in this article) as soon as possible. Caregivers are cautioned from turning the time out into a life lesson or lecture (eg, long drawn out conversations about why the child was in time out). These extensive explanations may unintentionally reinforce the original behavior. Sometimes, caregivers may need their own version of a "time out" and may benefit from taking 10 minutes away from the child to regulate themselves.

Ignore or distract from minor negative behavior

Selective attention or "active ignoring" is a parenting strategy that is very effective at reducing minor behavior or behaviors that are annoying to caregivers (eg, whining, tantrums, mocking, eye-rolling). This technique works best with younger children, but can be used at any age. It should never be used with unsafe behavior. By ignoring the behavior, parents can extinguish the behavior because the child is not receiving any attention (positive or negative).

That is not to say that ignoring is easy. In fact, it can be one of the hardest skills for parents to learn. With a typically developing child, ignoring means the parent has to totally disengage and take a time out–no talking, no eye contact, no physical response. Whining is a great example of a behavior that can be extinguished using this technique. However, parents must be warned that the child's behavior will initially escalate in response to the ignoring and parents need to stay the course. It is important that the caregiver continue to ignore the unwanted behavior and go about their business staying neutral and distracting themselves with other tasks, and the behavior will diminish. Eventually, children will figure out that the best way to be heard and receive attention from their caregiver is to interactive positively.

Sometimes, it is better to use distraction when possible (eg, blowing bubbles or telling a story). This particular strategy requires creativity and quick thinking on the part of the caregiver, and may not always be available if the caregiver is stressed or dysregulated themselves.

Self-efficacy

Self-efficacy refers to the belief that one has control over their own behavior or environment and is a skill that allows one to see a future for oneself where success is possible and that there are things a child can do that are within their control, thus creating a sense of hope. Pediatric medical providers can help caregivers to frame skills so that self-efficacy is promoted. Caregivers can be guided to challenge children to complete moderately difficult tasks, things that are just slightly out of reach for the skills of the child, which then, with support, reinforce a child's capacity and success and they learn that there are things they can do to control their environment and/or themselves. Allowing children to make a choice in simple situations ("Do you want to wear your blue sweater or red one?") instead of battling, and using natural consequences, which allow kids to see how their own choices impact outcomes, support the development of this process.

Medical providers can promote self-efficacy by encouraging caregivers to catch the chile being good; get curious, not furious; and educate.

Catch them being good

Positive reinforcement is powerful. When caregivers recognize a behavior that is to be encouraged, they should comment on it, and do so as specifically as possible. Ultimately, this demonstrates to a child their own success. Caregivers have a tendency to ignore children when they are demonstrating desired behaviors, but to respond or react to negative behavior. Affirming good behavior through positive attention can be a very powerful tool. Examples include:

- "I like how you are coloring. You are so focused."
- "I like how nicely you are playing with your sister."
- "Wow. Nice color choices. You are certainly creative."

Caregivers can catch siblings being nice to one other, a child playing quietly by themselves, or an adolescent being helpful. Specific, positive praise nurtures self-regulation and self-efficacy for all children.

Get curious, not furious

Every behavior has meaning and represents the thoughts and feelings that led to the expression of that behavior. By displaying curiosity about the child's behavior, rather than anger or frustration, caregivers can actually understand the thoughts and feelings behind the behaviors. When caregivers do this and engage the child in the process, the child develops regulation skills, problem solving, and executive function skills. Through understanding, the child's ability to self-regulate is increased, which promotes efficacy and, ultimately, mastery of these skills.

Educate

Rather than telling children what to do, modeling and teaching them what the caregiver would like the child to do is more effective. This process involves providing explanations and reasons for the behavior the caregiver wants to see. Caregivers cannot teach a "no" (eg, no fighting, no biting, etc). Telling a child not to do something may actually encourage a behavior by labeling and enhancing it. Therefore, caregivers should, instead, label and discuss the behaviors they want to see, rather than predominately discouraging the behaviors they do not want to see. Instead of "Stop that," say "In our house we color on paper" or "In our family we ask permission to use each other's toys."

Social Connectedness

Finally, social connectedness is the "railing along the staircase." These affiliative relationships outside the primary caregiving relationship support the child and caregiver all the way up the stairs. Consideration of the role of these supports, including family, friends, extended family, and the larger community, are critical components to build resilience in children, caregivers, and families. Caregivers need attachments and people who help to regulate them just as children do, and that comes from these social connections. By recognizing and identifying these other supports, it also helps the pediatric medical provider.

Every child and family needs a team of support, which includes the medical provider, but extends outside the pediatric office, particularly in times of need. Identifying this support network can be done through social network mapping–helping the caregiver to identify who they can call at various times throughout the day for support (eg, "You may feel like you are alone, but who would you call in the middle of the night?" and "Who would you call the next morning, or the next afternoon?" and "Who are the people you recognize as the experts in your life and the life of your child [eg, teacher, clergy person]?")

Ultimately what the pediatric medical provider offers

A confident expectation for success. The pediatric medical provider has a unique opportunity to promote attachment at every visit. We can project to the caregiver a confident expectation that they can effectively support their child, foster secure attachment, and help the child to achieve these necessary skills. This confident expectation of success is thus supported in the caregiver, and the caregiver can then project this to the child. In fact, this is an integral component of even the simplest, everyday interactions medical providers have with families. Up all night with a fussy child with a fever, a caregiver comes to the pediatric medical provider frightened and concerned that there is something very wrong with the child. The diagnosis of an ear infection and provision of advice to address it with supportive care at home comes with this confident expectation for recovery. That confident expectation provides safety and security for the caregiver, decreases their stress response, and allows them to feel confident that the child will recover as well. The child's fears can then be calmed by the caregiver. This pattern is repeated with all sorts of diagnoses, and child resilience is no exception. Supporting the caregiver's ability to help the child build resilience creates the space, confidence, and ability for the caregiver to do just that!

Disclosure

The authors have nothing to disclose.

References

[1] Traub F, Boynton-Jarrett R. Modifiable resilience factors to childhood adversity for clinical pediatric practice. Pediatrics 2017;139(5):e20162569.
[2] Garner AS, Shonkoff JP, Committee on Psychosocial Aspects of Child and Family Health, et al. Early childhood adversity, toxic stress, and the role of the pediatrician: translating developmental science into lifelong health. Pediatrics 2012;129(1):e224–31.
[3] Masten AS. Ordinary magic. Resilience processes in development. Am Psychol 2001;56(3):227–38.
[4] Manyena B, O'Brien G, O'Keefe P, et al. Disaster resilience: a bounce back or bounce forward ability? Local Environment: The International Journal of Justice and Sustainability 2011;16(5):417–24.
[5] Duft B, Stafford BS, Zeanah CH. Attachment disorders. Handbook of preschool mental health: development, disorders, and treatment. New York: The Guilford Press; 2017. p. 219–41.
[6] National Scientific Council on the Developing Child. Young children develop in an environment of relationships. Harvard University, Center on the Developing Child. Waltham (MA): Brandeis University; 2004.
[7] Shonkoff J. The timing and quality of early experiences combine to shape brain architecture: working paper No. 5. Cambridge (MA): National Scientific Council on the Developing Child; 2007.
[8] ACEs Pediatric healthcare toolkit. Available at: http://www.cascobaycan.org/cbcwp/wp-content/uploads/2015/12/2017ACEsToolkit.pdf. Accessed November 19, 2019.
[9] Hazan C, Shaver P. Romantic love conceptualized as an attachment process. J Pers Soc Psychol 1987;52(3):511–24.
[10] Allen JG. Restoring mentalizing in attachment relationships: treating trauma with plain old therapy. Arlington (VA): American Psychiatric Publishing; 2013.
[11] Attune. The Merriam-Webster.com Dictionary Web site. 2019. Available at: www.merriam-webster.com/dictionary/attune. Accessed November 29, 2019.
[12] Baylin J, Hughes DA. The neurobiology of attachment-focused therapy: enhancing connection & trust in the treatment of children & adolescents (Norton series on interpersonal neurobiology). New York: WW Norton & Company; 2016.
[13] Bretherton I. The origins of attachment theory: John Bowlby and Mary Ainsworth. Developmental Psychology 1992;28(5):759–75.

[14] Ainsworth MDS. Infancy in Uganda: infant care and the growth of love. Baltimore (MD): Johns Hopkins Press; 1967.
[15] Debiec J, Sullivan RM. The neurobiology of safety and threat learning in infancy. Neurobiol Learn Mem 2017;143:49–58.
[16] Allen JG, Fonagy P, Bateman AW. Mentalizing in clinical practice. Washington, DC: American Psychiatric Pub; 2008.
[17] Forkey H. Putting your trauma lens on. Pediatr Ann 2019;48(7):e269–73.
[18] Network TNCTS. Resource Parent Curriculum (RPC) online. 2011. Available at: https://www.nctsn.org/resources/resource-parent-curriculum-rpc-online. Accessed November 19, 2019.
[19] Fonagy P. On tolerating mental states: theory of mind in borderline personality. Bull Anna Freud Centre 1989;12(2):91–115.
[20] Jurkovic GJ. Lost childhoods: the plight of the parentified child. New York: Routledge; 2014.
[21] Blaustein ME, Kinniburgh KM. Treating traumatic stress in children and adolescents: how to foster resilience through attachment, self-regulation, and competency. New York: Guilford Publications; 2018.
[22] Paul HA. Treating trauma and traumatic grief in children and adolescents. In: Cohen JA, Mannarino AP, Deblinger E, editors. Treating trauma and traumatic grief in children and adolescents. (2nd Edition). New York: Taylor & Francis; 2017 xviii+ 356.
[23] Jellinek M, Patel BP, Froehle MC. Bright futures in practice: mental health. Arlington (VA): National Center for Education in Maternal and Child Health; 2002.
[24] Haydon AaN-T. Communicating scientific findings about adolescence and self-regulation: challenges and opportunities, Vol. 78. Washington, DC: Office of Planning Research and Evaluation AfCaF, U.S. Department of Health and Human Services; 2015.
[25] Blaustein M, Kinniburgh K. Treating traumatic stress in children and adolescents: how to foster resilience through attachment, self-regulation and competency. 2nd edition. New York: The Guilford Press; 2019.
[26] DiGiovanni S, Frances RH, Lawton A, et al. ACEs (adverse childhood experiences/trauma) pediatric healthcare toolkit. Portland (ME): Maine Medical Center; 2017.

Advances in Pediatrics 67 (2020) 29–46
ADVANCES IN PEDIATRICS

Meningococcal Infections in Children and Adolescents

Update and Prevention

Rebecca C. Brady, MD

Division of Infectious Diseases, Department of Pediatrics, Cincinnati Children's Hospital Medical Center, University of Cincinnati College of Medicine, 3333 Burnet Avenue, MLC 6014, Cincinnati, OH 45229-3039, USA

Keywords

• *Neisseria meningitidis* • Meningococcal disease • Meningococcemia • Meningitis • Immunization

Key points

- *Neisseria meningitidis* is a leading cause of sepsis and meningitis in young children and adolescents.
- Invasive meningococcal disease should be suspected when an individual presents with fever and a petechial rash, signs of meningitis, or shock.
- Prompt administration of a third-generation cephalosporin and early supportive therapy for shock improve outcomes in invasive meningococcal disease.
- Complement component deficiencies and anatomic or functional asplenia increase risk for invasive meningococcal disease.
- Meningococcal conjugate ACWY and new meningococcal B vaccines are important strategies for the prevention of meningococcal disease.

INTRODUCTION

A previously healthy 4-year-old boy presents to the emergency department with fever, altered mental status, prolonged capillary refill, and scattered petechiae on his legs. Despite intravenous ceftriaxone and vancomycin, aggressive fluid resuscitation and inotropic support, he dies within 8 hours. His blood and cerebrospinal fluid (CSF) cultures grow *Neisseria meningitidis.* In this article, the microbiology, epidemiology, clinical manifestations, diagnosis, treatment, and prevention of this devastating infection are reviewed.

E-mail address: rebecca.brady@cchmc.org

https://doi.org/10.1016/j.yapd.2020.03.007
0065-3101/20/

MICROBIOLOGY

N meningitidis is a gram-negative diplococcus (Fig. 1) that is divided into 13 serogroups based on the type of polysaccharide capsule [1–4]. Serogroups A, B, C, Y, and W are most commonly associated with disease [3]. The capsule enables the bacterium to resist host phagocytosis and complement-mediated lysis [5,6]. Another important virulence factor is lipooligosaccharide (LOS) endotoxin in the outer membrane of the cell envelope. Release of LOS triggers cytokine and chemokine cascades, leading to inflammation and septic shock [2,7].

Humans are the only known reservoir for *N meningitidis* [2]. The bacterium colonizes the nasopharyngeal tract and can be transmitted to close contacts by respiratory droplets [3]. Disease occurs when the bacteria invade the epithelia and enter the bloodstream, leading to systemic infection [8].

EPIDEMIOLOGY

Meningococcal disease occurs worldwide but rates are influenced by the geographic variation of circulating serogroups, environmental factors (eg, crowded living conditions, passive or active cigarette smoking), host factors (eg, age, malnutrition, immunodeficiency), and vaccination and other prevention strategies [2,9,10]. For most persons, nasopharyngeal carriage of *N meningitidis* is a natural immunizing process that generates a serum bactericidal antibody response to protect against infection with the same serogroup [8]. In the absence of protective antibodies, invasive meningococcal disease is more likely. Anatomic or functional asplenia is associated with impaired antibody production [6]. Complement components, especially the terminal

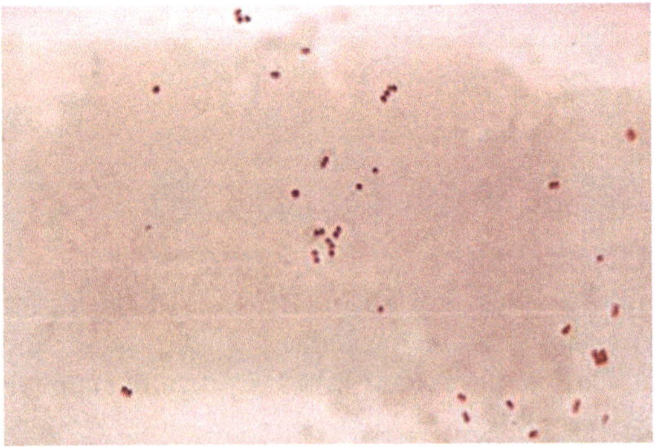

Fig. 1. The micrograph depicts the presence of aerobic gram-negative *N meningitidis* diplococcal bacteria (magnification ×1150; meningococcal disease is an infection caused by a bacterium called *N meningitidis* or the meningococcus. The meningococcus lives in the throat of 5%–10% of healthy people. Rarely, it can cause serious illness, such as meningococcal or blood infection). Source: Public Health Image Library Photo ID 6423. (*From* Centers for Disease Control and Prevention. Meningococcal Photos. In: Meningococcal Disease. Available at: https://www.cdc.gov/meningococcal/about/photos.html. Accessed November 14, 2019.)

membrane attack complex, mediate killing of *N meningitidis* and therefore individuals with congenital or acquired complement deficiencies have increased susceptibility to meningococcal disease [11].

Serogroup A is found in Africa, particularly in the "meningitis belt" between Senegal and Ethiopia (Fig. 2) [11]. Serogroup W has been associated with the Hajj pilgrimage to Mecca in Saudi Arabia [12]. Serogroups B and C account for most of the disease in Europe [13]. In North America, serogroups B, C, and Y predominate [6].

The annual incidence of meningococcal disease in the United States has ranged from 0.11 to 1.5 cases per 100,000 persons (Fig. 3) [14]. The incidence began to decline in 1995, which preceded the addition of the meningococcal conjugate vaccine to the recommended immunization schedule for adolescents in 2005 [3,11,15,16]. In 2017, there were about 350 total cases reported, with an incidence rate of 0.11 cases per 100,000 persons [14]. Potential explanations for this decrease include natural immunity within the population, changes in behavioral risk factors (such as decreases in smoking), and decreased virulence of circulating meningococcal strains [3,15,16].

Fig. 4 shows the incidence rates (per 100,000 persons) of meningococcal disease by age group in the United States from 2008 to 2017 [14]. The peak incidence was in the first 4 years of life, and a second peak occurred in those 15 to 24 years. Fig. 5 shows the incidence rates (per 100,000 persons) of serogroup B

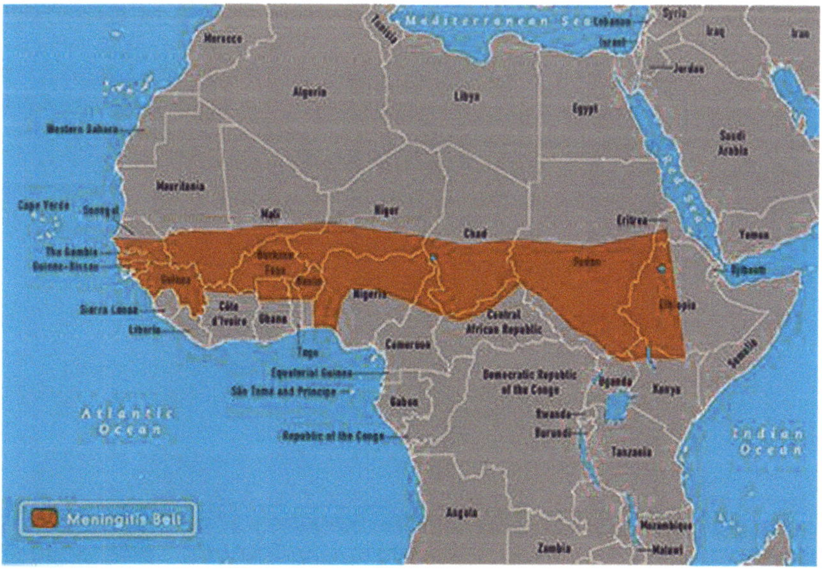

Fig. 2. The area in orange is the "meningitis belt" of sub-Saharan Africa where *N meningitidis* serogroup A is endemic. (*From* Centers for Disease Control and Prevention. Meningococcal disease. In: The Pink Book: Epidemiology and Prevention of Vaccine-Preventable Diseases. Atlanta, GA: Centers for Disease Control and Prevention; 2015. p. 238.)

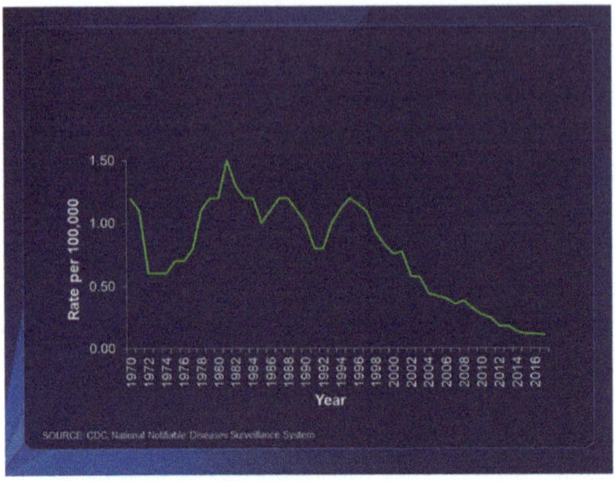

Fig. 3. Incidence rates (per 100,000 persons) of meningococcal disease in the United States by year from 1970 to 2017. The incidence rate began declining in 1995; it reached a historic low of 0.11 in 2017. (*From* Centers for Disease Control and Prevention. Meningococcal Disease Surveillance. In: Meningococcal Disease. Available at: https://www.cdc.gov/meningococcal/surveillance/index.html. Accessed November 14, 2019.)

disease compared with serogroups A, C, W, and Y by age group [14]. About 60% of meningococcal disease in infants less than 1 year was caused by serogroup B. Serogroups C, Y, and W (all covered by the meningococcal conjugate vaccine) accounted for about 66% of disease among those aged ≥11 years. By 2017, among those ≥11 years , only 42% of meningococcal disease was caused by serogroups C, Y, and W [14]. Meningococci have the capacity to

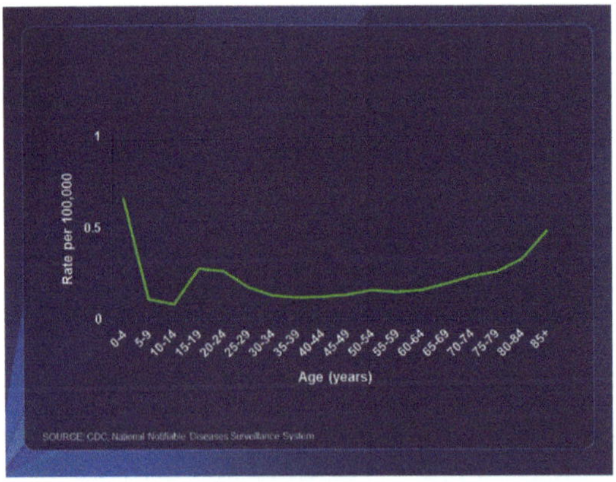

Fig. 4. Incidence rates (per 100,000 persons) of meningococcal disease by age group from 2008 to 2017. Infants, adolescents, and young adults have the highest rates of meningococcal disease in the United States. (*From* Centers for Disease Control and Prevention. Meningococcal Disease Surveillance. In: Meningococcal Disease. Available at: https://www.cdc.gov/meningococcal/surveillance/index.html. Accessed November 14, 2019.)

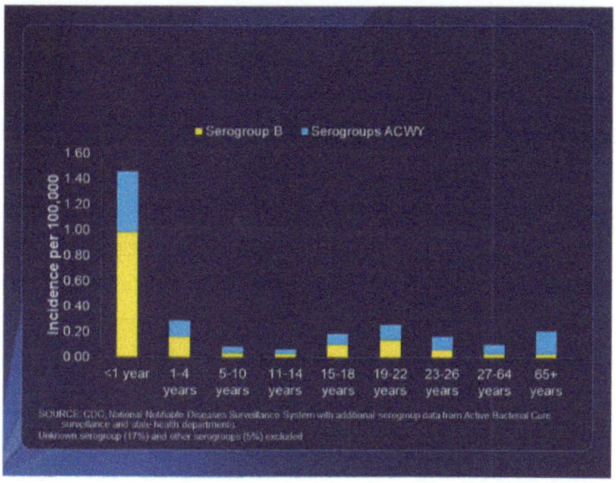

Fig. 5. Incidence rates (per 100,000 persons) of meningococcal disease due to serogroup B compared with serogroups A, C, W, and Y by age group from 2008 to 2017. Unknown serogroup (17%) and other serogroups (5%) are excluded. (*From* Centers for Disease Control and Prevention. Meningococcal Disease Surveillance. In: Meningococcal Disease. Available at: https://www.cdc.gov/meningococcal/surveillance/index.html. Accessed November 14, 2019.)

exchange the genetic material responsible for capsule production and thereby switch from serogroup C to B or vice versa [17], but the extent to which serogroup switching occurs in response to vaccination remains to be determined [1].

In the United States, *N meningitidis* is the leading cause of bacterial meningitis in children aged 11 to 17 years [3]. Most cases are sporadic and occur in the winter, often within 2 to 3 weeks after onset of influenza activity [3,11].

Less than 2% of meningococcal cases in the United States are associated with outbreaks [11,18]. Recently, several outbreaks of serogroup B meningococcal disease have been reported on college campuses [19–22]. Outbreaks have also been reported among child care center attendees, military recruits, and men who have sex with men [3,23].

CLINICAL MANIFESTATIONS

Invasive meningococcal disease may initially present with fever, headache, and myalgia, mimicking common viral illnesses [2,6,24]. Progression is often rapid, with the median time from onset of symptoms to hospital admission estimated at less than 22 hours in 1 study [24]. About 50% of cases result only in meningitis and the remainder are manifested as either sepsis (meningococcemia) or both sepsis and meningitis [1,3,11,15].

The signs and symptoms of meningococcal meningitis include irritability in younger children [6], and neck stiffness, headache, vomiting, and altered level of consciousness in older individuals [1]. Clinically, meningococcal meningitis is indistinguishable from other causes of acute bacterial meningitis [25].

Early signs of meningococcal sepsis may include fever, weakness, pallor or mottling, or cold hands and feet [26,27]. The rash may begin as macules or papules that become petechial (nonblanching) within hours [6]. Other viral infections (eg, Epstein-Barr virus, enterovirus, and measles), Rocky Mountain spotted fever, and severe sepsis attributable to other bacteria may result in a similar rash [3,24]. Disseminated intravascular coagulation, purpura fulminans leading to gangrene (Fig. 6), and multiorgan failure ensue quickly [2,4]. Adrenal hemorrhage leads to adrenal insufficiency, referred to as the Waterhouse-Friderichsen syndrome [9]. The overall case-fatality rate for meningococcemia is about 15% [3]. Risk factors for mortality include coma, hypotension, leukopenia, thrombocytopenia, and absence of meningitis [3,28]. Up to 20% of survivors have long-term sequelae, including loss of a limb, hearing loss, and neurologic disability [3,11].

A postinfectious, inflammatory syndrome, manifested by fever, arthritis, and vasculitis, occurs in less than 10% of cases [26]. This syndrome is due to the deposition of antigen-antibody complexes, begins a few days after treatment, and resolves spontaneously within 2 weeks [29]. Nonsteroidal anti-inflammatory drugs may provide relief of symptoms [26].

DIAGNOSIS

The finding of pleocytosis and gram-negative diplococci within neutrophils on cerebrospinal fluids (CSFs) provides a rapid and accurate presumptive diagnosis of meningococcal meningitis [30]. A positive culture of blood, CSF, a skin scraping of a petechial lesion, or other sterile site is considered the gold standard for diagnosis [6,31]. Blood cultures are positive in 40% to 75% and CSF cultures in 90% of those not pretreated with antibiotics [2,6,32]. Once *N meningitidis* is identified, the isolate should be submitted to a reference laboratory for serogrouping for epidemiologic purposes [2].

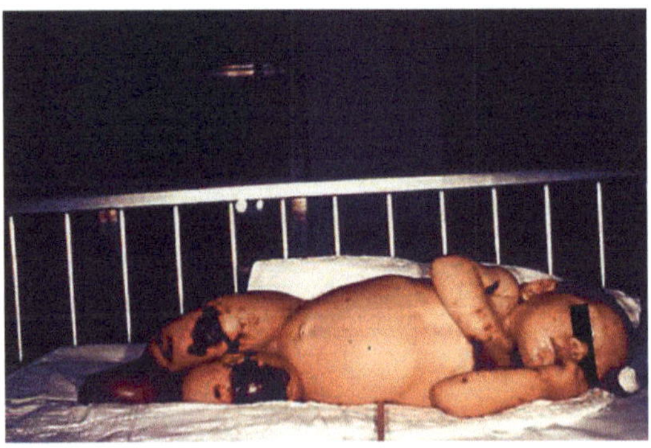

Fig. 6. Four-month-old baby girl with gangrene of the hands and lower extremities due to meningococcemia. Source: Public Health Image Library Photo ID (# 1335). (*From* Centers for Disease Control and Prevention. Meningococcal Photos. In: Meningococcal Disease. Available at: https://www.cdc.gov/meningococcal/about/photos.html. Accessed November 14, 2019.)

Latex agglutination (LA) tests to detect meningococcal polysaccharide types in CSF were developed more than 20 years ago [3]. LA is less sensitive than polymerase chain reaction (PCR) assays. The serogroup B polysaccharide may cross-react with K1 *Escherichia coli* capsular polysaccharide [2,33]. Therefore, LA has been replaced by PCR except in settings (eg, sub-Saharan Africa) where PCR is not available.

Multiplex PCR assays, which permit simultaneous testing for meningococci, pneumococci, *Haemophilus influenzae* type b, and other organisms, are useful in rapidly establishing the cause of meningitis [34]. Their sensitivity and specificity approach 100% for detection of serogroups A, B, C, W, and Y [3]. PCR performance is not affected by previous antibiotic administration.

Box 1 reviews the 2015 Centers for Disease Control and Prevention (CDC) surveillance case definitions for invasive meningococcal disease [31].

Box 1: Centers for Disease Control and Prevention surveillance case definitions for invasive meningococcal disease

Confirmed case

A clinically compatible case and isolation of *N meningitidis* from a usually sterile site, for example:

- Blood
- CSF
- Synovial fluid
- Pleural fluid
- Pericardial fluid
- Isolation from skin scraping of petechial or purpuric lesion

OR

Detection of *N meningitidis*-specific nucleic acid in a specimen obtained from a normally sterile body site (eg, blood or CSF), using a validated PCR assay

Probable case

A clinically compatible case with EITHER a positive result of antigen test OR immunohistochemistry of formalin-fixed tissue

Suspect case

- A clinically compatible case and gram-negative diplococci in any sterile fluid, such as CSF, synovial fluid, or scraping from a petechial or purpuric lesion
- Clinical purpura fulminans without a positive culture

Adapted from Centers for Disease Control and Prevention. Meningococcal Disease (*Neisseria meningitidis*) 2015 Case Definition. Available at: https://wwwn.cdc.gov/nndss/conditions/meningococcal-disease/case-definition/2015.

TREATMENT

Antibiotic therapy

Invasive meningococcal disease is a medical emergency. Early antibiotic therapy combined with management of shock improves outcomes [1,2]. In settings where hospital transfer may be delayed (eg, in developing countries), ceftriaxone is administered intramuscularly once the diagnosis is suspected [2,35]. Once in the emergency department, the priority is to obtain blood specimens for culture and immediately administer antibiotics [6]. The drug of choice is a third-generation cephalosporin, such as ceftriaxone [36]. In cases of suspected bacterial meningitis, ceftriaxone is usually combined with vancomycin to also cover penicillin-resistant and ceftriaxone-resistant *Streptococcus pneumoniae* until the causative bacteria has been identified [37]. If antibiotics are administered before obtaining CSF, other CSF parameters (eg, increased white blood cell count, increased protein, or low glucose) are still helpful in assessing for central nervous system involvement [6]. Meningococci in CSF are killed within 4 hours after intravenous ceftriaxone therapy so the culture may be negative if the lumbar puncture is delayed [38].

Once *N meningitidis* has been identified from the blood or CSF culture, vancomycin is discontinued. Antimicrobial susceptibility testing is often not routinely performed and rapid assays used for other bacteria (eg, Etests, disk diffusion, and automated systems) are not standardized for *N meningitidis* [39]. In addition, the clinical significance of intermediate susceptibility to penicillin is unknown [2]. Third-generation cephalosporins have excellent in vitro and in vivo effectiveness and achieve optimal CSF concentrations to treat meningococcal infections [40]. Therefore, they are the antibiotics of choice. Ceftriaxone clears nasopharyngeal carriage after 1 dose [3]. Duration is 5 to 7 days for meningococcemia and meningococcal meningitis [6]. For hospitalized patients, droplet precautions are recommended until 24 hours after initiation of effective antibiotic therapy [3]. In suspected cases without a positive culture (eg, clinical purpura fulminans) [31], treatment with ceftriaxone is usually continued unless an alternative diagnosis is established.

Supportive care

The initial management of invasive meningococcal disease is often best accomplished in the intensive care unit [2]. Meningococcal LOS endotoxin induces cytokine and chemokine cascades that lead to vascular collapse and shock [2,7]. Early and rapid fluid resuscitation and inotropic support reduce mortality [41]. Dialysis or hemofiltration may be needed to compensate for kidney injury and to reduce the massive edema from fluid resuscitation [2]. Meningitis may be complicated by raised intracranial pressure or the syndrome of inappropriate antidiuretic hormone secretion [36]. Disseminated intravascular coagulation is managed by treating the underlying infection [2]. Stress doses of hydrocortisone are required if shock is accompanied by adrenal insufficiency [42]. Once the patient with purpura fulminans and gangrene is stabilized and a clear line of demarcation between viable and nonviable tissue is present, necrotic tissue is debrided [43].

Follow-up care

All children with bacterial meningitis should have their hearing assessed either before or shortly after hospital discharge [2]. Those who have lost a limb need physical and occupational therapy [44]. Even those who seem well at the completion of antibiotic therapy are at risk for impaired school performance and behavioral problems [3] so close follow-up with their primary care clinician is encouraged. Providers should also consider whether to evaluate the patient for an underlying condition (eg, a complement component deficiency) that increases the risk for invasive meningococcal disease [45].

PREVENTION

Care of people exposed to cases of invasive meningococcal disease

Postexposure chemoprophylaxis

N meningitidis can be transmitted from a person to his/her close contacts through droplets from the respiratory tract [3]. Household contacts of cases have 500 to 800 times the rate of disease for the general population [11].

The goal of postexposure chemoprophylaxis is to identify close contacts of patients with meningococcal disease who may have acquired the organism, and then promptly administer antibiotics to eradicate nasopharyngeal colonization before infection ensues [46]. Throat and nasopharyngeal cultures are not recommended because waiting for their results unnecessarily delays chemoprophylaxis initiation [3]. Chemoprophylaxis is recommended for household contacts and other high-risk contacts (eg, child care or preschool contact at any time during 7 days before the onset of illness) [47]. Even if the contact has previously received meningococcal vaccines, chemoprophylaxis is still provided because the currently licensed vaccines are not 100% effective [3]. Ideally, chemoprophylaxis should be initiated less than 24 hours after the index patient is identified but may still be effective if started within 2 weeks of exposure [47].

Antibiotics for chemoprophylaxis

Effective antibiotics for meningococcal chemoprophylaxis achieve bactericidal levels in the tears and saliva, and thus eradicate colonization [46]. Penicillin, ampicillin, and chloramphenicol do not meet this criterion [2,3]. Recommended chemoprophylaxis for high-risk contacts is provided in Table 1 [3,48]. Chemoprophylaxis with these recommended agents is 90% to 95% effective [49]. If the index patient does not receive at least 1 dose of ceftriaxone or cefotaxime during treatment of invasive meningococcal disease, then chemoprophylaxis should be received before hospital discharge to eradicate carriage [3].

Postexposure vaccination

When an outbreak is caused by a vaccine-preventable serogroup, local public health authorities may also recommend a meningococcal vaccine containing the outbreak serogroup [3]. For outbreaks caused by serogroups A, C, W, and Y, the preferred vaccine in persons aged 2 months to 55 years is the meningococcal conjugate ACWY vaccine (Tables 2 and 3) [3,50–54]. For a

Table 1
Recommended antibiotic chemoprophylaxis for high-risk contacts

Antibiotic	Dose	Comments
Rifampin	Children <1 mo: 5 mg/kg, orally, every 12 h for 2 d Children ≥1 mo: 15–20 mg/kg (maximum 600 mg), orally, every 12 h for 2 d	Nor recommended for pregnant women Can stain soft contact lens Can interfere with efficacy of oral contraceptives and some seizure prevention and anticoagulant medications
Ceftriaxone	Children <15 y: 125 mg, single intramuscular (IM) dose Children ≥15 y and adults: 250 mg, single IM dose	Recommended for prophylaxis in pregnant women
Ciprofloxacin	20 mg/kg (maximum 500 mg) single oral dose	Not recommended routinely for persons <18 y Not recommended for pregnant or lactating women Use only if fluoroquinolone-resistant strains of *N meningitidis* have not been identified in the local community
Azithromycin	10 mg/kg (maximum 500 mg) single oral dose	*Not* recommended routinely; equivalent to rifampin for eradication of meningococci from the nasopharynx, but data are limited

Adapted from Bilukha OO, Rosenstein N; National Center for Infectious Diseases, Centers for Disease Control and Prevention (CDC). Prevention and control of meningococcal disease. Recommendations of the Advisory Committee on Immunization Practices (ACIP). MMWR Recomm Rep 2005;54(RR-7):1-21; and American Academy of Pediatrics. Meningococcal infections. In: Kimberlin DW, Brady MT, Jackson MA, Long SS, editors. Red Book: 2018 Report of the Committee on Infectious Diseases. 31st edition. Itasca, IL: American Academy of Pediatrics; 2018. p. 550-61.

Table 2
Meningococcal conjugate ACWY vaccines

Name	Trade name	Licensed	Carrier protein	Age group approval
MenACWY-D	Menactra (Sanofi Pasteur, Swiftwater, PA)	2005	Diphtheria toxoid protein	9 mo through 55 y
MenACWY-CRM	Menveo (Novartis Vaccines and Diagnostics, Inc, Cambridge, MA)	2010	Diphtheria CRM_{197} protein	2 mo through 55 y

Data from Cohn AC, MacNeil JR, Clark TA, et al. Centers for Disease Control and Prevention. Prevention and control of meningococcal disease: recommendations of the Advisory Committee on Immunization Practices (ACIP). MMWR Recomm Rep 2013;62(RR-02):1-28.

Table 3
Recommended MenACWY immunization schedule and intervals for people at increased risk of invasive meningococcal disease

Age	Subgroup	Primary immunization
2 through 23 mo	Persistent complement component deficiency, including eculizumab use	MenACWY-CRM • Dose 1 at age 8 wk: 4-dose series at 2, 4, 6, and 12 mo • Dose 1 at age 7–23 mo: 2-dose series (dose 2 at least 12 wk after dose 1 and after the first birthday) MenACWY-D • Age 9–23 mo: 2 doses at least 12 wk apart • Must be administered at least 4 wk after completion of the pneumococcal 13-valent conjugate vaccine (PCV13) series
	Anatomic or functional asplenia or human immunodeficiency virus (HIV) infection	MenACWY-CRM • Dose 1 at age 8 wk: 4-dose series at 2, 4, 6, and 12 mo • Dose 1 at age 7–23 mo: 2-dose series (dose 2 at least 12 wk after dose 1 and after the first birthday) MenACWY-D • Age 9–23 mo: not recommended
	Travel in countries with hyperendemic or epidemic disease	MenACWY-CRM • Dose 1 at age 8 wk: 4-dose series at 2, 4, 6, and 12 mo • Dose 1 at age 7–23 mo: 2-dose series (dose 2 at least 12 wk after dose 1 and after the first birthday) MenACWY-D • Age 9–23 mo: 2 doses (dose 2 may be administered as early as 8 wk after dose 1) • Must be administered at least 4 wk after completion of PCV13 series
24 mo or older (through 55 y) and not immunized previously	Persistent complement component deficiency, including eculizumab use, anatomic or functional asplenia, or HIV infection	MenACWY-CRM: 2-dose series at least 8 wk apart MenACWY-D: 2-dose series at least 8 wk apart (must be administered at least 4 wk after completion of PCV13 series)
	Travel in countries with hyperendemic or epidemic disease	MenACWY-D or MenACWY-CRM: 1 dose (MenACWY-D must be administered at least 4 wk after completion of the PCV13 series)

Adapted from Centers for Disease Control and Prevention. Recommended child and adolescent immunization schedule for ages 18 years or younger, United States, 2019. Available at: https://www.cdc.gov/vaccines/schedules/hcp/imz/child-adolescent.html. Accessed November 22, 2019.

meningococcal serogroup B outbreak, either of the 2 licensed serogroup B vaccines may be administered to persons 10 years and older (Table 4) [3,54–58].

Prophylaxis during eculizumab therapy
Eculizumab (Soliris, Alexion Pharmaceuticals) is a terminal complement inhibitor that is licensed in the United States for the treatment of paroxysmal nocturnal hemoglobinuria and atypical hemolytic uremic syndrome (aHUS) [59]. It is also used for the therapy for thrombotic microangiopathy among allogeneic stem cell transplant recipients. Terminal complement inhibition impairs in vitro opsonophagocytic killing of meningococci in whole blood and leads to a 1000- to 2000-fold increased incidence of meningococcal disease [60]. To mitigate this increased risk, the Advisory Committee on Immunization Practices recommends that eculizumab recipients receive both the quadrivalent meningococcal conjugate (MenACWY) and serogroup B (MenB) meningococcal vaccines [3,54].

Between 2008 and 2016, 16 cases of meningococcal disease were identified in eculizumab recipients in the United States [61]. Fourteen patients had documentation of receipt of at least 1 dose of meningococcal vaccine before disease onset. Eleven of these 16 cases were caused by nongroupable *N meningitidis*, which is not included in the currently licensed vaccines. Therefore, antibiotic prophylaxis (eg, penicillin) is recommended for the duration of eculizumab treatment (lifelong for many patients) [3,59]. If eculizumab is stopped, antibiotic prophylaxis is continued until immunocompetence is restored to potentially reduce the risk for meningococcal disease.

Meningococcal polysaccharide vaccines

Meningococcal polysaccharide vaccines for serogroups A, C, and later Y and W, were introduced in the 1970s and 1980s in military and civilian

Table 4
Meningococcal B vaccines

Name	Trade name	Licensed	Antigens	Age group approval
MenB-FHbp	Trumenba (Wyeth, Philadelphia, PA)	2014	Two recombinant lipidated factor H-binding protein (FHbp) variants	10 through 25 y
MenB-4C	Bexsero (Novartis Vaccines and Diagnostics, Inc, Cambridge, MA)	2015	1. One recombinant lipidated FHbp variant 2. Neisserial adhesion A (NadA) 3. Neisserial heparin binding antigen 4. PorA-containing outer membrane vesicle preparation	10 through 25 y

Adapted from MacNeil JR, Rubin L, Folaranmi T, et al. Use of serogroup B meningococcal vaccines in adolescents and young adults: recommendations of the Advisory Committee on Immunization Practices, 2015. MMWR Morb Mortal Wkly Rep 2015;64(41):1171-6.

populations and for control of disease outbreaks [62–64]. The meningococcal polysaccharide vaccines induce serum bactericidal antibodies, are safe, and are greater than 85% effective in older children and adults [2]. However, children less than 2 years cannot mount adequate immune responses to T-cell-independent polysaccharide antigens. Polysaccharide antigens also do not generate immunologic memory responses. Therefore, the meningococcal ACWY polysaccharide vaccine was discontinued in the United States in 2017 [65].

Meningococcal A, C, W, and Y conjugate vaccines

The successful introduction of capsular polysaccharide-protein conjugate vaccines for *H influenzae* type b [66] and *S pneumoniae* [37] fueled the development of meningococcal polysaccharide-protein conjugate vaccines. Conjugation leads to a T-cell-dependent immune response, which is protective in infants as young as 2 months [67]. This strategy reduces nasopharyngeal carriage of *N meningitidis*, decreases transmission risk, and provides herd immunity. In the United States, 2 meningococcal conjugate vaccines against serogroups A, C, W, and Y (MenACWY) are licensed and available (see Table 2) [3,54].

MenACWY conjugate vaccine is recommended for all adolescents as a 2-dose series with the first dose administered at age 11 to 12 years and a booster dose at age 16 years [54]. For those 13 to 15 years who have not been previously vaccinated, the first dose should be administered now and a second dose should be administered at age 16 to 18 years with a minimum interval of 8 weeks between the 2 doses. For those starting vaccination at ≥16 years, only 1 dose is required.

Common adverse events after MenACWY vaccination include pain, erythema and swelling at the injection site, headache, and fatigue [3]. Syncope can occur after any vaccination and is most common among adolescents and young adults [68]. Adolescents should receive the vaccine while seated or lying down and remain in this position for at least 15 minutes after immunization to prevent syncope. If syncope develops, the patient should be observed until symptoms resolve. Syncope after vaccine receipt is not a contraindication to future doses.

Box 2 lists people who are at increased risk of invasive meningococcal disease [3,54]. Table 3 provides the recommended immunization schedule and intervals for these individuals [54]. If the individual remains at increased risk, then booster doses are needed and their spacing depends on the age of the receipt of the first dose. For those who receive the first dose between 2 months and 6 years, a booster dose is administered 3 years after the first dose and then repeated every 5 years thereafter. For those receiving the first dose at age ≥7 years, a booster is administered 5 years after the first dose and then repeated every 5 years thereafter. MenACWY-D vaccine should be administered either before or at the same time as DTaP (diphtheria, tetanus, and acellular pertussis) vaccine when both are indicated.

Box 2: Individuals at increased risk of invasive meningococcal disease

Have persistent complement component deficiencies (eg, C3, C5-C9, properdin, or factor D or factor H or receiving eculizumab)

Have anatomic or functional asplenia (including sickle cell anemia)

Have human immunodeficiency virus infection

Travel to or are residents of countries where meningococcal disease is hyperendemic or epidemic, including countries in the African meningitis belt or during the Hajj

Are at risk during a community outbreak attributable to a vaccine serogroup

Are laboratory workers routinely exposed to isolates of *N meningitidis*

Adapted from Centers for Disease Control and Prevention. Recommended child and adolescent immunization schedule for ages 18 years or younger, United States, 2019. Available at: https://www.cdc.gov/vaccines/schedules/hcp/imz/child-adolescent.html. Accessed November 22, 2019.

Meningococcal B vaccines

Serogroup B *N meningitidis* is also a leading cause of meningococcal disease in infants, young children, and adolescents in many countries [6,13]. Because the serogroup B polysaccharide resembles the human neural cell adhesion molecule and other human antigens, it is poorly immunogenic and carries a potential risk of autoimmunity [2,69]. Therefore, attention focused on other semiconserved surface proteins for use as vaccine antigens. Using "reverse vaccinology" strategies [2,70], 2 serogroup B meningococcal (MenB) vaccines were licensed in the United States in 2014 and 2015, respectively (see Table 4) [3,54].

MenB vaccine is recommended for those at increased risk of invasive meningococcal disease (see Box 2) [54]. For MenB-FHbp, a 3-dose series should be administered at 0, 1 to 2, and 6 months; for MenB-4C, 2 doses are administered at least 1 month apart [54]. MenB-FHbp and MenB-4C are not interchangeable; the same product should be used for all doses in a series.

For adolescents not at increased risk of invasive meningococcal disease, MenB vaccine may be administered based on shared clinical decision making [56,58]. The preferred age is 16 to 18 years. For MenB-FHbp, a 2-dose series is recommended with at least 6 months between the 2 doses [54]. If the second dose is administered earlier than 6 months, administer a third dose at least 4 months after dose 2. For MenB-4C, 2 doses are administered at least 1 month apart.

MenB vaccination activates complement, and therefore, complement-mediated processes (eg, hemolysis) may temporarily worsen after vaccine receipt in patients receiving eculizumab for treatment of aHUS [3]. Otherwise, adverse events are similar to other vaccines.

Potential differences between the 2 MenB vaccines in immunogenicity and breadth of coverage are not completely known [58]. Vaccine effectiveness and duration of protection are still being evaluated [3]. For the most current recommendations, clinicians should consult the CDC Advisory Committee on Immunization Practice guidelines.

SUMMARY

N meningitidis is a leading cause of sepsis and meningitis in young children and adolescents [6]. Prompt initiation of antibiotic therapy and early correction of shock improve outcomes [1,2]. Antibiotic prophylaxis of close contacts mitigates the spread of disease [46]. Routine vaccination of all adolescents with MenACWY vaccine and of high-risk individuals with both MenACWY and MenB vaccines are important strategies for controlling meningococcal disease [54]. The MenB vaccine may also be administered to healthy 16- to 18-year-old individuals using shared decision making [56,58]. Studies of the effect of these vaccines on disease incidence and severity continue [3].

Disclosure

The author has nothing to disclose.

References

[1] Rosenstein NE, Perkins BA, Stephens DS, et al. Meningococcal disease. N Engl J Med 2001;344(18):1378–88.
[2] Stephens DS, Apicella MA. Neisseria meningitidis. In: Bennett JE, Dolin R, Blaser MJ, editors. Mandell, Douglas, and Bennett's principles and practice of Infectious diseases. 8th edition. Philadelphia: WB Saunders; 2015. p. 2425–45.
[3] American Academy of Pediatrics. Meningococcal infections. In: Kimberlin DW, Brady MT, Jackson MA, et al, editors. Red book: 2018 report of the committee on infectious diseases. 31st edition. Itasca (IL): American Academy of Pediatrics; 2018. p. 550–61.
[4] Centers for Disease Control and Prevention. Meningococcal Photos. In: Meningococcal Disease. Available at: https://www.cdc.gov/meningococcal/about/photos.html. Accessed November 14, 2019.
[5] Rouphael NG, Stephens DS. *Neisseria meningitidis*: biology, microbiology, and epidemiology. Methods Mol Biol 2012;799:1 20.
[6] Vaz LE. Meningococcal disease. Pediatr Rev 2017;38:158–69.
[7] Zughaier SM, Tzeng YL, Zimmer SM, et al. *Neisseria meningitidis* lipooligosaccharide structure-dependent activation of the macrophage CD14/Toll-like receptor 4 pathway. Infect Immun 2004;72:371–80.
[8] Stephens DS. Uncloaking the meningococcus: dynamics of carriage and disease. Lancet 1999;353:941–2.
[9] Stephens DS, Greenwood B, Brandtzaeg P. Epidemic meningitis, meningococcaemia, and *Neisseria meningitidis*. Lancet 2007;369:2196–210.
[10] Harrison LH, Trotter CL, Ramsey ME. Global epidemiology of meningococcal disease. Vaccine 2009;27(Suppl 2):B51–63.
[11] Centers for Disease Control and Prevention. Meningococcal disease. In: Hamborsky J, Kroger A, Wolfe S, editors. The pink book: epidemiology and prevention of vaccine-preventable diseases. Atlanta (GA): Centers for Disease Control and Prevention; 2015. p. 231–46.
[12] Aguilera JF, Perrocheau A, Meffre C, et al. Outbreak of serogroup W135 meningococcal disease after the Hajj pilgrimage, Europe, 2000. Emerg Infect Dis 2002;8:761–7.
[13] Schwartz B, Moore PS, Broome CV. Global epidemiology of meningococcal disease. Clin Microbiol Rev 1989;2(Suppl):S118–24.

[14] Centers for Disease Control and Prevention. Meningococcal Disease Surveillance. In: Meningococcal Disease. Available at: https://www.cdc.gov/meningococcal/surveillance/index.html. Accessed November 14, 2019.
[15] Rosenstein NE, Perkins BA, Stephens DS, et al. The changing epidemiology of meningococcal disease in the United States, 1992-1996. J Infect Dis 1999;180(6):1894–901.
[16] Harrison LH. Epidemiological profile of meningococcal disease in the United States. Clin Infect Dis 2010;50(Suppl 2):S37–44.
[17] Swartley JS, Marfin AA, Edupuganti S, et al. Capsule switching of *Neisseria meningitidis.* Proc Natl Acad Sci U S A 1997;94:271–6.
[18] Brooks R, Woods CW, Benjamin DK Jr, et al. Increased case-fatality rate associated with outbreaks of *Neisseria meningitidis* infection, compared with sporadic meningococcal disease, in the United States, 1994-2002. Clin Infect Dis 2006;43(1):49–54.
[19] Mandal S, Wu HM, MacNeil JR, et al. Prolonged university outbreak of meningococcal disease associated with a serogroup B strain rarely seen in the United States. Clin Infect Dis 2013;57(3):344–8.
[20] McNamara LA, Shumate AM, Johnsen P, et al. First use of a serogroup B meningococcal vaccine in the US in response to a university outbreak. Pediatrics 2015;135:798–804.
[21] Soeters HM, McNamara LA, Whaley M, et al. Serogroup B meningococcal disease outbreak and carriage evaluation at a college—Rhode Island, 2015. MMWR Morb Mortal Wkly Rep 2015;64:606–7.
[22] Biswas HH, Han GS, Wendorf K, et al. Notes from the field: outbreak of serogroup B meningococcal disease at a university—California, 2016. MMWR Morb Mortal Wkly Rep 2016;65(20):520–1.
[23] Centers for Disease Control and Prevention. Notes from the field: serogroup C invasive meningococcal disease among men who have sex with men-New York City, 2010-2012. MMWR Morb Mortal Wkly Rep 2013;61(51–52):1048.
[24] Thompson MJ, Ninis N, Perera R, et al. Clinical recognition of meningococcal disease in children and adolescents. Lancet 2006;367(9508):397–403.
[25] Feigin RD, Dodge PR. Bacterial meningitis: newer concepts of pathophysiology and neurologic sequelae. Pediatr Clin North Am 1976;23(3):541–56.
[26] Pace D, Pollard AJ. Meningococcal disease: clinical presentation and sequelae. Vaccine 2012;30(Suppl 2):B3–9.
[27] Kornelisse RF, Hazelzet JA, Hop WC, et al. Meningococcal septic shock in children: clinical and laboratory features, outcome, and development of a prognostic score. Clin Infect Dis 1997;25:640–6.
[28] Castellanos-Ortega A, Delgado-Rodríguez M, Llorca J, et al. A new prognostic scoring system for meningococcal septic shock in children. Comparison with three other scoring systems. Intensive Care Med 2002;28(3):341–51.
[29] Goedvolk CA, von Rosenstiel IA, Bos AP. Immune complex associated complications in the subacute phase of meningococcal disease: incidence and literature review. Arch Dis Child 2003;88:927–30.
[30] Dunbar SA, Eason RA, Musher DM, et al. Microscopic examination and broth culture of cerebrospinal fluid in diagnosis of meningitis. J Clin Microbiol 1998;36:1617–20.
[31] Centers for Disease Control and Prevention. Meningococcal Disease (*Neisseria meningitidis*) 2015 Case Definition. Available at: https://wwwn.cdc.gov/nndss/conditions/meningococcal-disease/case-definition/2015. Accessed November 15, 2019.
[32] Hoyne AL, Brown RH. Seven hundred and twenty seven meningococcic cases; an analysis. Ann Intern Med 1948;28:248–59.
[33] Finlay FO, Witherow H, Rudd PT. Latex agglutination in bacterial meningitis. Arch Dis Child 1995;73:160–1.
[34] Corless CE, Guiver M, Borrow R, et al. Simultaneous detection of *Neisseria meningitidis, Haemophilus influenzae*, and *Streptococcus pneumoniae* in suspected cases of meningitis and septicemia using real-time PCR. J Clin Microbiol 2001;39:1553–8.

[35] Hahné SJ, Charlett A, Purcell B, et al. Effectiveness of antibiotics given before admission in reducing mortality from meningococcal disease: systemic review. BMJ 2006;332(7553): 1299–303.
[36] National Institute for Health and Care Excellence (NICE). Meningitis (bacterial) and meningococcal septicaemia in under 16s: recognition, diagnosis, and management (Clinical Guideline 102), London, UK. 2010. Available at: http://www.nice.org.uk/CG102. Accessed November 15, 2019.
[37] American Academy of Pediatrics. Pneumococcal infections. In: Kimberlin DW, Brady MT, Jackson MA, et al, editors. Red book: 2018 report of the committee on infectious diseases. 31st edition. Itasca (IL): American Academy of Pediatrics; 2018. p. 639–51.
[38] Kanegaye JT, Soliemanzadeh P, Bradley JS. Lumbar puncture in pediatric bacterial meningitis: defining the time interval for recovery of cerebrospinal fluid pathogens after parenteral antibiotic pretreatment. Pediatrics 2001;108:1169–74.
[39] Terranella A, Beekmann SE, Polgreen PM, et al. Practice patterns of infectious disease physicians for management of meningococcal disease. Pediatr Infect Dis J 2012;31:e208–12.
[40] Goldwater PN. Cefotaxime and ceftriaxone cerebrospinal fluid levels during treatment of bacterial meningitis in children. Int J Antimicrob Agents 2005;26:408–11.
[41] Pollard AJ, Britto J, Nadel S, et al. Emergency management of meningococcal disease. Arch Dis Child 1999;80:290–6.
[42] Campsall PA, Laupland KB, Niven DJ. Severe meningococcal infection: a review of epidemiology, diagnosis, and management. Crit Care Clin 2013;29:393–409.
[43] Wheeler JS, Anderson BJ, De Chalain TM. Surgical interventions in children with meningococcal purpura fulminans a review of 117 procedures in 21 children. J Pediatr Surg 2003;38:597–603.
[44] Buysse CM, Oranje AP, Zuidema E, et al. Long-term skin scarring and orthopaedic sequelae in survivors of meningococcal septic shock. Arch Dis Child 2009;94:381–6.
[45] Hoare S, El-Shazali O, Clark JE, et al. Investigation for complement deficiency following meningococcal disease. Arch Dis Child 2002;86:215–7.
[46] Hoeprich PD. Prediction of antimeningococcic chemoprophylactic efficacy. J Infect Dis 1971;123:125–33.
[47] Centers for Disease Control and Prevention. Control and prevention of meningococcal disease: recommendations of the Advisory Committee on Immunization Practices (ACIP). MMWR Recomm Rep 1997;46(RR-5):1–10.
[48] Bilukha OO, Rosenstein N, National Center for Infectious Diseases, Centers for Disease Control and Prevention (CDC). Prevention and control of meningococcal disease. Recommendations of the Advisory Committee on Immunization Practices (ACIP). MMWR Recomm Rep 2005;54(RR-7):1–21.
[49] Gardner P. Clinical practice. Prevention of meningococcal disease. N Engl J Med 2006;355:1466–73.
[50] Centers for Disease Control and Prevention. Infant meningococcal vaccination: Advisory Committee on Immunization Practices (ACIP) recommendations and rationale. MMWR Morb Mortal Wkly Rep 2013;62:52–4.
[51] Cohn AC, MacNeil JR, Clark TA, et al. Centers for Disease Control and Prevention. Prevention and control of meningococcal disease: recommendations of the Advisory Committee on Immunization Practices (ACIP). MMWR Recomm Rep 2013;62(RR-02):1–28.
[52] MacNeil JR, Rubin L, McNamara L, et al. Meningitis and Vaccine Preventable Diseases Branch, Division of Bacterial Diseases, National Center for Immunization and Respiratory Diseases, CDC. Use of MenACWY-CRM vaccine in children aged 2 through 23 months at increased risk for meningococcal disease: recommendations of the Advisory Committee on Immunization Practices, 2013. MMWR Morb Mortal Wkly Rep 2014;63:527–30.
[53] American Academy of Pediatrics Committee on Infectious Diseases. Updated recommendations on the use of meningococcal vaccines. Pediatrics 2014;134(2):400–3.

[54] Centers for Disease Control and Prevention. Recommended child and adolescent immunization schedule for ages 18 years or younger, United States, 2019. Available at: https://www.cdc.gov/vaccines/schedules/hcp/imz/child-adolescent.html. Accessed November 22, 2019.
[55] Folaranmi T, Rubin L, Martin SW, et al. Centers for Disease Control and Prevention. Use of serogroup B meningococcal vaccines in persons aged ≥10 years at increased risk for serogroup B meningococcal disease: recommendations of the Advisory Committee on Immunization Practices, 2015. MMWR Morb Mortal Wkly Rep 2015;64(22):608–12.
[56] MacNeil JR, Rubin L, Folaranmi T, et al. Use of serogroup B meningococcal vaccines in adolescents and young adults: recommendations of the Advisory Committee on Immunization Practices, 2015. MMWR Morb Mortal Wkly Rep 2015;64(41):1171–6.
[57] Patton ME, Stephens D, Moore K, et al. Updated recommendations for use of MenB-FHbp serogroup B meningococcal vaccine—Advisory Committee on Immunization Practices, 2016. MMWR Morb Mortal Wkly Rep 2017;66(19):509–13.
[58] American Academy of Pediatrics Committee on Infectious Diseases. Recommendations for serogroup B meningococcal vaccine for persons 10 years and older. Pediatrics 2016;138(3):e20161890.
[59] Food and Drug Administration. Soliris product insert. Silver Spring (MD): US Department of Health and Human Services, Food and Drug Administration; 2017. Available at: https://www.accessdata.fda.gov/drugsatfda_docs/label/2017/125166s417lbl.pdf. Accessed November 4, 2019.
[60] Konar M, Granoff DM. Eculizumab treatment and impaired opsonophagocytic killing of meningococci by whole blood from immunized adults. Blood 2017;130(7):891–9.
[61] McNamara LA, Topaz N, Wang X, et al. High risk for invasive meningococcal disease among patients receiving eculizumab (Soliris) despite receipt of meningococcal vaccine. MMWR Morb Mortal Wkly Rep 2017;66(27):734–7.
[62] Artenstein MS, Gold R, Zimmerly JG, et al. Prevention of meningococcal disease by group C polysaccharide vaccine. N Engl J Med 1970;282:417–20.
[63] Makela PH, Käyhty H, Weckström P, et al. Effect of group-A meningococcal vaccine in army recruits in Finland. Lancet 1975;2:883–6.
[64] Lepow ML, Beeler J, Randolph M, et al. Reactogenicity and immunogenicity of a quadrivalent combined meningococcal polysaccharide vaccine in children. J Infect Dis 1986;154:1033–6.
[65] Pasteur S. Sanofi Pasteur statement on the discontinuation of meningococcal polysaccharide vaccine, groups A, C, Y and W-135 combined. Available at: http://www.news.sanofi.us/Sanofi-Pasteur-Statement-on-the-Discontinuation-of-Meningococcal-Polysaccharide-Vaccine-Groups-A-C-Y-and-W-135-Combined. Accessed November 23, 2019.
[66] Robbins JB, Schneerson R, Anderson P, et al. The 1996 Albert Lasker Medical Research Awards. Prevention of systemic infections, especially meningitis, caused by *Haemophilus influenzae* type b. Impact on public health and implications for other polysaccharide-based vaccines. JAMA 1996;276:1181–5.
[67] Pichichero ME. Protein carriers of conjugate vaccines: characteristics, development, and clinical trials. Hum Vaccin Immunother 2013;9:2505–23.
[68] Centers for Disease Control and Prevention. Syncope after vaccination—United States, January 2005-July 2007. MMWR Morb Mortal Wkly Rep 2008;57(17):457–60.
[69] Stephens DS. Outer-membrane-vesicle vaccines: old but not forgotten. Lancet Infect Dis 2011;11:421–2.
[70] Richmond PC, Marshall HS, Nissen MD, et al. Safety, immunogenicity, and tolerability of meningococcal serogroup B bivalent recombinant lipoprotein 2086 vaccine in healthy adolescents: a randomised, single-blind, placebo-controlled, phase 2 trial. Lancet Infect Dis 2012;12:597–607.

Advances in Pediatrics 67 (2020) 47–56

ADVANCES IN PEDIATRICS

Pediatric Hepatitis C

Sara Kathryn Smith, MD

Department of Pediatric Gastroenterology, Hepatology, and Nutrition, University of California, San Francisco, 550 16th Street, 5th Floor, Mail Code 0136, San Francisco, CA 94158, USA

Keywords

• Viral hepatitis • Hepatitis • Hepatitis C • HCV • Direct acting antivirals

Key points

- Hepatitis C virus infection in children differs from that in adults.
- Vertical transmission is the most common mode of transmission of hepatitis C virus in children in developed countries.
- Although spontaneous resolution may occur, most children progress to chronic hepatitis C virus infection.
- New oral, interferon-free drug regimens have revolutionized the treatment of hepatitis C virus infection and are now approved for use in children over 3 years of age.

INTRODUCTION

Optimal care of children with viral hepatitis requires that clinical practice integrates the most recent updates in diagnosis, prevention, and treatment. Although primary viral infections of the liver were first recognized by Hippocrates in 460 to 375 BC, it was not until the early 1990s that clinicians were able to use advances in understanding these viruses to alter outcomes. We have been successful in developing methods to detect these infections early, rapidly, and accurately and this has led to significant changes in epidemiology of viral hepatitis. Hepatitis C virus (HCV) accounts for approximately 15% to 20% of cases of acute hepatitis and about 50% to 80% of patients will develop chronic infection. Most of our understanding of HCV infection is derived from the study of HCV infection in adults. We now understand that HCV infection in children differs from HCV infection acquired later in life. Differences exist for modes of transmission, rates of spontaneous clearance, progression of fibrosis, potential duration of chronic

*Corresponding author.

https://doi.org/10.1016/j.yapd.2020.03.008
0065-3101/20/Published by Elsevier Inc.

infection, and available treatment options. More recently, the development of oral direct-acting antiviral agents (DAA) for the treatment of HCV has led to dramatic reductions in the prevalence and incidence of the virus and the possibility of future eradication of the virus.

VIRUS CHARACTERISTICS

HCV is a hepatotropic RNA virus of the genus *Hepacivirus* in the Flaviviridae family, originally cloned in 1989 as causative agent of non-A, non-B hepatitis [1]. HCV is a positive sense, single-stranded enveloped RNA virus approximately 9600 nucleotides in length. HCV genomic RNA is packaged by core protein and enveloped by a lipid bilayer containing 2 viral glycoproteins (E1 and E2) to form the virion [2].

There are 6 major HCV genotypes (numbered 1–6), each with variations in the nucleotide sequence. Despite the nucleotide sequence variance among genotypes, all currently recognized HCV genotypes are hepatotropic and pathogenic. Genotypes vary in geographic distribution with genotype 1 being the most common in North America (HCV1a) and Europe (HCV1b). Genotypes 1, 2, and 3 all have worldwide distribution, genotype 4 is found mainly in North Africa and the Middle East, genotype 5 in South Africa, and genotype 6 in Asia [3].

INFECTIVITY

Viral entry into the host cell comprises a complex series of interactions, including attachment, entry, and fusion. The HCV lifecycle starts with attachment of a virion to specific receptors on hepatocytes. Cellular receptors and entry factors for HCV include scavenger receptor class B type 1 and CD81, along with tight junction proteins, claudin-1 and occludin. Receptor tyrosine kinases epidermal growth factor receptor, ephric receptor A1, and Niemann-Pick C1-like cholesterol absorption receptor have been recently identified as entry factors [4]. After attachment, HCV is internalized into target cells via a pH-dependent and clathrin-mediated endocytosis, after which the nucleocapsid is released into the cytoplasm. Once the virus is released into the cytoplasm, the virus is then uncoated and HCV genomic RNA is used both for polyprotein translation and replication in the cytoplasm. Replication takes place within a “replication complex” containing viral nonstructural proteins and cellular proteins. The HCV assembly and release process has not been fully elucidated; however, it involves the very low-density lipoprotein synthesis and secretion machinery. The HCV virion is a lipoviroparticle with a lipid composition with apolipoprotein E and/or apolipoprotein B, which are crucial for the infectious virus assembly [4].

TRANSMISSION

HCV is a blood-borne illness. In the United States, most infections are acquired via injection drug use, particularly in settings where needles are shared. Sexual transmission has also been reported, mainly in men having sex with men, with an increased risk in those with a concomitant human immunodeficiency virus

Box 1: Children for whom HCV screening is recommended

Children who are or were injection drug users

Children who are HIV positive

Children who have ever required dialysis

Children with unexplained or chronically elevated aminotransferase levels

Children born to mothers with documented HCV infection

Children who are sexual partners of an HCV-infected person

Children from region with high prevalence of HCV infections

Adapted from Recommendations for prevention and control for hepatitis C virus (HCV infection and HCV-related chronic disease. Centers for disease control and prevention. MMWR Recomm Rep 1998;47(RR019):1-39; and Mack CL, Gonzalez-Peralta RP, Gupta N, et al. NASPHGAN practice guidelines: diagnosis and management of hepatitis C infection in infants, children, and adolescents J Pediatr Gastroenterol Nutr 2012;54(6):838-55.

(HIV) infection with multiple sex partners. In low-income countries, HCV infection is associated with unsafe injection and procedures in medical facilities without adequate infection control practices [5].

In the past, HCV infection in children was considered a transfusion related disease; since the initiation of blood screening practices, no new cases of transfusion-transmitted HCV infection have been documented since 1994. In children, the primary mode of transmission is vertical, from infected mother to child, and accounts for about 60% of cases [6]. Rates of transmission are about 5% to 10% from HCV RNA positive mono-infected and HIV co-infected mothers, respectively [7]. Higher rates of vertical transmission are seen in women with a history of injection drug abuse and women with peripheral mononuclear blood cell infection. Possible risk factors for transmission include invasive prenatal testing, prolonged rupture of the membranes, and invasive obstetric procedures, such as fetal scalp monitoring. Studies have been mixed regarding an association between maternal viral load and vertical transmission. There are no methods to prevent vertical transmission of HCV; however, early identification and effective treatment in young women with HCV before conception is vital. The majority of new HCV infections occur among adolescents and young adults who are injection drug users, specifically those who have been victims of the oral opioid abuse epidemic and have transitioned to opioid and heroin injection. Other potential methods of transmission include tattooing and body piercing [5]. Testing is indicated for children at risk for HCV. Box 1 outlines screening guidelines for HCV in children.

EPIDEMIOLOGY

HCV treatments first became available in the early 1990s and, since then, the incidence rate of HCV infection has markedly decreased. Despite the decrease in incidence, deaths from the long-term sequalae of HCV infection, including cirrhosis, hepatocellular carcinoma, and liver failure, continue to increase. There are approximately 115 million cases of HCV infection in the world. Eleven million of these cases are in patients youngers than 11 years of age, of which 5 million are viremic [3].

According to National Health and Nutrition Examination Survey data, in the United States, antibodies to HCV are present in approximately 0.2% of children ages 6 to 12 years and 0.4% of children ages 12 to 19 years [8]. It is unknown what proportion of children who are HCV antibody positive are also HCV RNA positive; however, based on studies in adults, the estimate is around 75% to 80%.

CLINICAL ASPECTS AND PATHOGENESIS

Spontaneous clearance of acute HCV infection can occur within 6 months of infection in around 20% of adult patients in the absence of treatment [9]. In children infected via vertical transmission, somewhere between 20% and 45% of these spontaneously clear the infection in the first 4 years of life [10–12]. Spontaneous resolution can occur up to 7 or 8 years of age, but is rare after 3 years of age [12–14]. Anywhere from 6% to 12% of children with chronic HCV infection will clear the virus [15], with the remainder of these children developing chronic infection [16]. Infected children have a low risk of progression of disease and only about 5% develop significant liver disease in childhood. Viral characteristics, including genotype, and host factors have an impact on rates of spontaneous clearance in vertically transmitted HCV infection [10].

The incubation period for HCV infection ranges from 2 weeks to 6 months, and more than three-quarters of HCV-infected children are asymptomatic [11,12] with normal to mildly increased serum alanine aminotransferase levels. About 15% of children with HCV infection exhibit nonspecific signs and symptoms, such as hepatomegaly, fever, lethargy, anorexia, nausea, vomiting, abdominal pain, and arthralgias, among other symptoms [17].

Chronic HCV infection is defined the same in children and adults, that is, evidence of active viral infection with detectable RNA for at least 6 months. Compared with adults that exhibit more rapid disease progression, evidence of disease progression in children is typically only seen in those who have been infected for 10 years or more [18,19]. The difference is accounted for by additional risk factors and comorbidities present in the adult population, including alcohol consumption and HIV co-infection. Cirrhosis has been reported in 1% to 2% of children with chronic HCV [13] and liver transplantation has been performed in children with advanced liver disease from chronic HCV [20].

Certain biologic factors can affect the natural history of infection in children. There is an increased risk of more severe disease in patients with a history of childhood cancer [21], co-infection with hepatitis B or HIV, obesity [22], and congenital anemias requiring chronic transfusions [22]. There are also well-documented effects on the natural history of chronic HCV in children with risky behaviors, such as intravenous drug use and alcohol use in teenagers [23].

DIAGNOSIS

The diagnosis of HCV infection starts with an initial screening for evidence of past or current infection with an HCV serologic assay (antibody or antibody/antigen) followed by nucleic acid testing for HCV RNA to confirm the presence of HCV viremia. Because the immunoassay tests are easy to perform, automated, reliable, and inexpensive, antibody-based tests are generally recommended for screening. The disadvantage of antibody-based tests is that they cannot distinguish between acute and chronic infection. Third-generation enzyme immunoassays detecting antibodies against core protein and nonstructural proteins 3, 4, and 5 become positive around 6 to 8 weeks after infection is acquired. During the acute phase of HCV infection, anti-HCV IgG antibodies generally do not return positive and serum HCV RNA should be used to determine infection (Table 1). HCV RNA can be detected in plasma using rapid polymerase chain reaction testing as early as 1 to 2 weeks after exposure and weeks before antibody testing become positive [24]. Anti-HCV IgM is not recommended and does not distinguish between acute and chronic HCV infection.

Anti-HCV IgG crosses the placenta, so testing for anti-HCV is not useful in children less than 18 months of age [25]. Children older than 18 months with positive anti-HCV IgG should then be tested for serum HCV RNA to determine if they have active infection. Infants who have positive serum HCV RNA before 18 months should have repeat testing after 12 months of age to confirm the presence of active HCV infection. Spontaneous clearance may occur up to 4 years of age in children acquiring HCV infection via vertical transmission; therefore, confirmation of chronic HCV can be postponed until after this age. HCV genotyping is useful in guiding antiviral therapy and duration of therapy, especially now in the era of DAA therapy.

MONITORING

Annual evaluations should be done on children with chronic HCV infection who are not receiving therapy. Laboratory monitoring includes a complete blood count with platelets, serum aminotransferases, bilirubin (total and direct), albumin, HCV RNA levels, and prothrombin time/international normalized ratio (if cirrhosis is present). A liver biopsy is generally not performed, except in cases when the result will affect management decisions or in the setting of unexplained clinical hepatic decompensation in a previously stable patient with chronic HCV infection [26]. Hepatocellular carcinoma in children with chronic HCV infection is rare; however, in children with significant liver disease, abdominal ultrasound examination and serum alpha-fetoprotein should be considered for surveillance of hepatocellular carcinoma [26–28].

TREATMENT

Before the development of oral DAAs for the treatment of HCV infection, the only available treatment regimen for children with HCV infection included pegylated interferon (Peg-IFN) and ribavirin. IFN-alpha is a cytokine that acts by

Table 1
Interpretation of HCV testing

Anti-HCV IgG Ab	HCV RNA (RT-PCR)	Interpretation
Positive	Positive	Acute or chronic depending on clinical context
Positive	Negative	Resolution of infection or acute infection during low level viremia*
Negative	Positive	Early acute infection Chronic infection in setting of immunosuppression False-positive HCV RNA

Abbreviations: Ab, antibody; PT-PCR, reverse transcriptase polymerase chain reaction.
*If HCV RNA is negative and remains negative when repeated 6 mo later, chronic HCV infection has been ruled out.

increasing antigen presentation of viral peptides stimulating action of CD8-positive T cells and natural killer cells and inducing synthesis of key antiviral protein mediators [28]. Ribavirin, a guanosine analog, interrupts viral RNA synthesis by interfering with HCV RNA polymerase. Ribavirin is added to IFN-alpha treatment to increase the sustained virologic response (SVR) and decrease the rate of relapse and development of viral resistance [29]. Not only is Peg-IFN a weekly injection, but the combined treatment regimen of Peg-IFN and ribavirin had multiple adverse effects, including fever, headache, gastrointestinal symptoms, depression, neutropenia, hemolytic anemia, and growth suppression.

Oral DAAs are now the preferred treatment in adult patients with HCV and are fast becoming the preferred treatment in children. HCV RNA is translated into a single polyprotein that is cleaved into structural and nonstructural proteins using viral and cellular proteases. DAAs target these nonstructural proteins of HCV designated as NS2, NS3, NS4A, NS4B, NS5A, and NS5B. NS2 and NS3 are proteases; NS4A is a cofactor for NS3; NS4B causes changes in the cellular membrane to allow viral replication; NS5A is involved in regulation of viral replication; and NS5B is an RNA polymerase [30]. The combination of different classes of DAAs has been shown in adults to reduce the development of viral resistance and improved SVR rates. Studies have shown comparable pharmacokinetics and safety profiles in adult and adolescent populations with HCV infection. The use of fixed dose combination of ledipasvir/sofosbuvir and sofosbuvir with ribavirin was approved in 2017 for the treatment of chronic HCV infection in adolescents (ages 12–17) with genotypes 1, 4, 5, and 6 and genotypes 2 and 3, respectively. In August 2019, the US Food and Drug Administration approved the use of ledipasvir/sofosbuvir in children with HCV infection aged 3 years and older with genotype 1, 4, 5, or 6 without cirrhosis or with compensated cirrhosis and in those with genotype 1 with decompensated cirrhosis [31]. Sofosbuvir with ribavirin was also approved for use in children over the age of 3 with HCV genotypes 2 and 3 in August 2019. The US Food and Drug Administration approved the use of glecaprevir/

pibrentasvir for treatment of genotypes 1 to 6 in children ages 12 to 17 years with chronic HCV infection without cirrhosis in May 2019 [32]. The duration of treatment for DAA drug regimens range from 8 to 24 weeks and depend on genotype, previous treatment, hepatic compensation, and/or transplant status (Table 2). Trials using other combination DAAs in children with HCV are ongoing and early results are promising.

For younger children less than 3 years of age, the only approved treatment remains Peg-IFN and ribavirin for 24 to 28 weeks; however, international guidelines now recommend deferring treatment until children are eligible for treatment with DAAs. All children more than 3 years of age with chronic HCV infection, whether treatment naïve or treatment experienced, should be considered for DAA therapy for eradication of HCV infection. Studies to date have shown great efficacy with the use of DAAs in children and adolescents with chronic HCV, independent of age, treatment history, treatment duration, and degree of liver fibrosis. The safety profile of DAAs is also favorable in children and adolescents [16,33–35]. Peg-IFN and some DAAs are contraindicated in the use of decompensated cirrhosis [35,36]. The most common cited adverse effects with the use of DAAs in children are headache and fatigue.

The goal of treatment is to achieve SVR once treatment is discontinued. SVR is affected by age, viral load, fibrosis score, genotype, and compliance with therapy. In children, the aim of treatment is not only to cure HCV infection, but also to prevent the progression of HCV related liver disease and its complications. Therapy is considered successful when HCV RNA is undetectable in the blood

Table 2
Recommended oral treatment regimens for HCV infection in children[c]

Genotype	Duration	Regimen
1, 2, 3, 4, 5, or 6	8–16 wk[a]	Ages 12–17 ≥35 kg: glecaprevir 300 mg/pibrentasvir 120 mg once daily
1, 4, 5, or 6	12–24 wk[a]	Ages 3–17 <17 kg: 33.75 mg ledipasvir/150 mg sofosbuvir once daily 17 to <35 kg: 45 mg ledipasvir/200 mg sofosbuvir once daily ≥35 kg: 90 mg ledipasvir/400 mg sofosbuvir once daily
2,3	12–24 wk[a]	Ages 3–17 <17 kg: 150 mg sofosbuvir once daily + ribavirin[b] 17 to <35 kg: 200 mg sofosbuvir once daily + ribavirin[b] ≥35 kg: 400 mg sofosbuvir once daily + ribavirin[b]

[a]Duration depends on genotype, previous treatment, hepatic compensation, and/or transplant status.
[b]Dosing based on weight.
[c]Before starting therapy, patients should be tested for evidence of hepatitis B infection (current or prior).

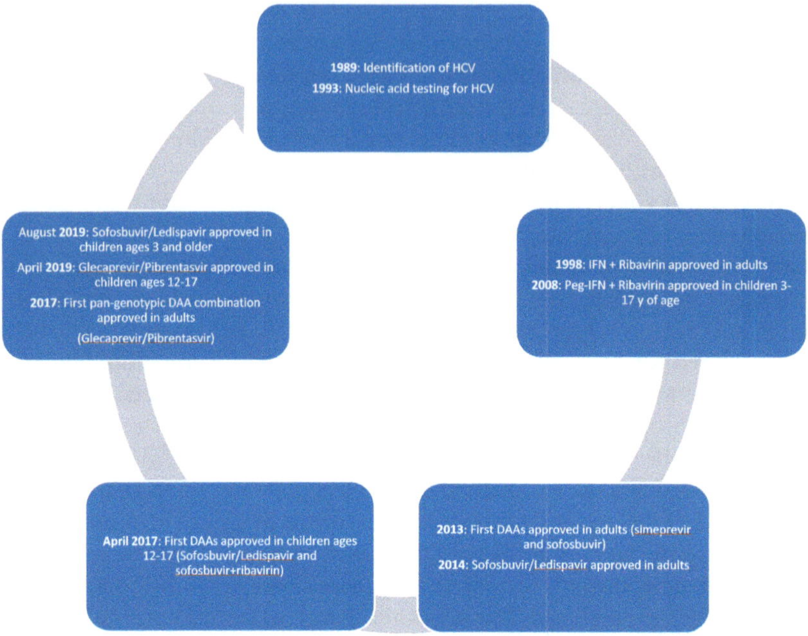

Fig. 1. Milestones in HCV research and treatment. (*Adapted from* Treatment of adolescents with chronic Hepatitis C virus infection: New regimen on the block. Hepato Commun 2018;2(11): 1289-1292.)

(the lower limit of detection is ≤15 IU/mL), 12 weeks after completion of DAA treatment or 24 weeks after completion of Peg-IFN and ribavirin treatment. The introduction of DAAs has revolutionized the treatment of HCV infection (Fig. 1) and increasing use will hopefully lead to a decrease in the incidence and prevalence of HCV infection and may also help to decrease new vertically and horizontally acquired pediatric HCV infections [37].

PREVENTION AND COUNSELING

Families of children and adolescents with chronic HCV should be counseled regarding the specific routes of transmission and recommendations to reduce transmission to others. Caution should be used when sharing toothbrushes, razors, nail clippers, and other tools that may become contaminated with blood from an infected user. For adolescents and older children, specific counseling should be given regarding avoidance of high-risk behaviors, such as self-tattooing, self-piercing, injection drug use, and having multiple sexual partners. At this time, a vaccine for HCV does not exist. Eradication of HCV infection will rely on continued development of oral drug treatment regimens and widespread institution of these regimens to decrease the prevalence, incidence, and transmission of HCV.

Disclosure

Neither author has any direct financial interest in subject matter or materials discussed in article or with a company making a competing product.

References

[1] Farci P. Choo QL, Kuo G, Weiner AJ, Overby LR, Bradley DW, Houghton M. Isolation of a cDNA clone derived from a blood-borne non-A, non-B viral hepatitis genome [science 1989;244:359–362]. J Hepatol 2002;36(5):582–5. Available at: http://www.sciencedirect.com/science/article/pii/S016882780200051X.

[2] Neumann AU, Lam NP, Dahari H, et al. Hepatitis C viral dynamics in vivo and the antiviral efficacy of interferon-alpha therapy. Science 1998;282(5386):103–7.

[3] El-Shabrawi MH, Kamal NM. Burden of pediatric hepatitis C. World J Gastroenterol 2013;19(44):7880–8.

[4] Kim CW, Chang KM. Hepatitis C virus: virology and life cycle. Clin Mol Hepatol 2013;19(1):17–25.

[5] Centers for Disease Control and Prevention. Hepatitis C. Available at: https://www.cdc.gov/hepatitis/hcv/index.htm. Accessed December 1, 2019.

[6] Ly KN, Jiles RB, Teshale EH, et al. Hepatitis C virus infection among reproductive-aged women and children in the united states, 2006 to 2014. Ann Intern Med 2017;166(11):775–82.

[7] Benova L, Mohamoud YA, Calvert C, et al. Vertical transmission of hepatitis C virus: systematic review and meta-analysis. Clin Infect Dis 2014;59(6):765–73.

[8] Denniston MM, Jiles RB, Drobeniuc J, et al. Chronic hepatitis C virus infection in the united states, national health and nutrition examination survey 2003 to 2010. Ann Intern Med 2014;160(5):293–300.

[9] Grebely J, Page K, Sacks-Davis R, et al. The effects of female sex, viral genotype, and IL28B genotype on spontaneous clearance of acute hepatitis C virus infection. Hepatology 2014;59(1):109–20.

[10] Resti M, Jara P, Hierro L, et al. Clinical features and progression of perinatally acquired hepatitis C virus infection. J Med Virol 2003;70(3):373–7.

[11] European Paediatric Hepatitis C Virus Network. Three broad modalities in the natural history of vertically acquired hepatitis C virus infection. Clin Infect Dis 2005;41(1):45–51.

[12] Bortolotti F, Verucchi G, Cammà C, et al. Long-term course of chronic hepatitis C in children: from viral clearance to end-stage liver disease. Gastroenterology 2008;134(7):1900–7. Available at: http://www.sciencedirect.com/science/article/pii/S0016508508004174.

[13] Jara P, Resti M, Hierro L, et al. Chronic hepatitis C virus infection in childhood: clinical patterns and evolution in 224 white children. Clin Infect Dis 2003;36(3):275–80.

[14] Rerksuppaphol S, Hardikar W, Dore GJ. Long-term outcome of vertically acquired and post-transfusion hepatitis C infection in children. J Gastroenterol Hepatol 2004;19(12):1357–62.

[15] Indolfi G, Mangone G, Bartolini E, et al. Hepatitis C viraemia after apparent spontaneous clearance in a vertically infected child. Lancet 2016;387(10031):1967–8.

[16] Vogt M, Lang T, Frösner G, et al. Prevalence and clinical outcome of hepatitis C infection in children who underwent cardiac surgery before the implementation of blood-donor screening. N Engl J Med 1999;341(12):866–70.

[17] Sokal E, Nannini P. Chapter 6.1. Pediatric chronic hepatitis B and C: 30 years of ESPGHAN clinical research and recommendations. J Pediatr Gastroenterol Nutr 2018;66 Suppl 1:S119–21. Available at: http://hdl.handle.net/2078.1/196761. Accessed December 1, 2019.

[18] Gonzalez-Peralta RP, Langham MR Jr, Andres JM, et al. Hepatocellular carcinoma in 2 young adolescents with chronic hepatitis C. J Pediatr Gastroenterol Nutr 2009;48(5):630–5.

[19] Guido M, Bortolotti F, Jara P, et al. Liver steatosis in children with chronic hepatitis C. Am J Gastroenterol 2006;101(11):2611–5.

[20] Rumbo C, Fawaz RL, Emre SH, et al. Hepatitis C in children: a quaternary referral center perspective. J Pediatr Gastroenterol Nutr 2006;43(2):209–16.

[21] Cesaro S, Bortolotti F, Petris MG, et al. An updated follow-up of chronic hepatitis C after three decades of observation in pediatric patients cured of malignancy. Pediatr Blood Cancer 2010;55(1):108–12.

[22] Delgado-Borrego A, Healey D, Negre B, et al. Influence of body mass index on outcome of pediatric chronic hepatitis C virus infection. J Pediatr Gastroenterol Nutr 2010;51:191–7.

[23] Page K, Hahn JA, Evans J, et al. Acute hepatitis C virus infection in young adult injection drug users: a prospective study of incident infection, resolution, and reinfection. J Infect Dis 2009;200(8):1216–26.

[24] Gupta E, Bajpai M, Choudhary A. Hepatitis C virus: screening, diagnosis, and interpretation of laboratory assays. Asian J Transfus Sci 2014;8(1):19–25.

[25] England K, Pembrey L, Tovo PA, et al, European Paediatric HCV Network. Excluding hepatitis C virus (HCV) infection by serology in young infants of HCV-infected mothers. Acta Paediatr 2005;94(4):444–50.

[26] Mack C, Gonzalez-Peralta R, Gupta N, et al. NASPGHAN practice guidelines: diagnosis and management of hepatitis C infection in infants, children, and adolescents. J Pediatr Gastroenterol Nutr 2012;54(6):838–55. Available at: http://ovidsp.ovid.com/ovidweb.cgi?T=JS&NEWS=n&CSC=Y&PAGE=fulltext&D=ovft&AN=00005176-201206000-00030. Accessed December 1, 2019.

[27] Strickland DK, Jenkins JJ, Hudson MM. Hepatitis C infection and hepatocellular carcinoma after treatment of childhood cancer. J Pediatr Hematol Oncol 2001;23(8):527–9. Available at: https://journals.lww.com/jpho-online/Fulltext/2001/11000/Hepatitis_C_Infection_and_Hepatocellular_Carcinoma.12.aspx.

[28] Pham YH, Rosenthal P. Chronic hepatitis C infection in children. Adv Pediatr 2016;63(1):173–94.

[29] Schwarz KB, Gonzalez-Peralta RP, Murray KF, et al. The combination of ribavirin and peginterferon is superior to peginterferon and placebo for children and adolescents with chronic hepatitis C. Gastroenterology 2011;140(2):450–8.e1.

[30] Bell TW. Drugs for hepatitis C: unlocking a new mechanism of action. ChemMedChem 2010;5(10):1663–5.

[31] Harvoni: ledipasvir and sofosbuvir FDA. Available at: https://www.accessdata.fda.gov/drugsatfda_docs/label/2019/212477s000lbl.pdf. Accessed December 1, 2019.

[32] FDA news release: FDA approves first treatment for all genotypes of hepatitis C in pediatric patients. Available at: https://www.fda.gov/news-events/press-announcements/fda-approves-first-treatment-all-genotypes-hepatitis-c-pediatric-patients. Accessed December 1, 2019.

[33] Balistreri WF, Murray KF, Rosenthal P, et al. The safety and effectiveness of ledipasvir-sofosbuvir in adolescents 12-17 years old with hepatitis C virus genotype 1 infection. Hepatology 2017;66(2):371–8.

[34] Wirth S, Rosenthal P, Gonzalez-Peralta RP, et al. Sofosbuvir and ribavirin in adolescents 12-17 years old with hepatitis C virus genotype 2 or 3 infection. Hepatology 2017;66(4):1102–10.

[35] Indolfi G, Ricci S. Treatment of adolescents with chronic hepatitis C virus infection: new regimen on the block. Hepatol Commun 2018;2(11):1289–92. Available at: https://www.ncbi.nlm.nih.gov/pubmed/30411074 https://www.ncbi.nlm.nih.gov/pmc/articles/PMC6211323/.

[36] Ghany MG, Strader DB, Thomas DL, et al. American Association for the Study of Liver Diseases. Diagnosis, management, and treatment of hepatitis C: an update. Hepatology 2009;49(4):1335–74.

[37] Leung DH, Wirth S, Yao BB, et al. Ombitasvir/paritaprevir/ritonavir with or without dasabuvir and with or without ribavirin for adolescents with HCV genotype 1 or 4. Hepatol Commun 2018;2(11):1311–9.

Advances in Pediatrics 67 (2020) 57–71

ADVANCES IN PEDIATRICS

Advances in Sickle Cell Disease Management

Elissa R. Engel, MD[a], Alexandra L. Howard, DO, MPH[a], Emily J. Ankus, BS[b], Juan Felipe Rico, MD[c,*]

[a]Department of Pediatrics, University of South Florida Morsani College of Medicine, 2 Tampa General Circle, Tampa, FL 33606, USA; [b]University of South Florida Morsani College of Medicine, 2 Tampa General Circle, 5th Floor, Tampa, FL 33606, USA; [c]Division of Hematology/Oncology, Department of Pediatrics, University of South Florida Morsani College of Medicine, Tampa, FL, USA

Keywords

• Sickle cell disease • Sickle cell anemia • Management • Screening • Infants • Children • Adolescents

Key points

- Sickle cell disease is associated with significant morbidity and a shortened life span.
- Screening for complications of sickle cell disease, such as pulmonary hypertension, renal disease, stroke, and neurocognitive decline, is important in pediatric patients because morbidity and mortality increase with age.
- Hydroxyurea, L-glutamine, crizanlizumab-tmca, and voxelotor are FDA approved for the treatment of sickle cell disease.
- Curative options being investigated for the treatment of sickle cell disease include bone marrow transplant and gene therapy.

INTRODUCTION

Sickle cell disease (SCD) is the most common inherited hemoglobinopathy in the United States. Approximately 100,000 Americans are affected, with the highest prevalence in African-Americans (about 1/365) and Hispanic-Americans (about 1/16,300) [1,2]. Internationally, the prevalence is highest in sub-Saharan Africa; more than 75% of individuals with SCD are born in this region [3]. Other areas with significant disease burden include Central

*Corresponding author. *E-mail address:* jrico@usf.edu

https://doi.org/10.1016/j.yapd.2020.03.001

America, the Caribbean, Brazil, Greece, Italy, the Middle East, and the Indian subcontinent [4].

Hemoglobin S (HbS), or sickle hemoglobin, arises from a point mutation in the ß-globin gene on chromosome 11. The point mutation causes glutamate to be substituted for valine at the sixth codon. In a deoxygenated state, unstable HbS molecules polymerize resulting in "sickling" of the red blood cells [5]. These sickled red blood cells can obstruct vasculature leading to tissue ischemia and pain. HbSS disease, the most common SCD variant, is transmitted to offspring in an autosomal-recessive manner. Thus, each parent must contribute a mutated ß-globin gene for their child to have HbSS disease. Other variants of SCD include sickle cell hemoglobin C (HbSC) and sickle cell β-thalassemia major (HbS/$ß^0$). SCD encompasses all variants of the disease with sickle cell anemia (SCA) used to describe the most severe forms. The US Preventive Services Task Force recommended universal newborn screening for SCD and this recommendation was implemented in all 50 states in 2008 [6]. This recommendation was given an "A" grade, meaning that "there is high certainty that the net benefit is substantial." If newborn screening results are suggestive of SCD confirmatory testing with hemoglobin electrophoresis should be performed before 2 months of age.

Within the first few months of life infants are protected from the effects of SCD because of a high concentration of fetal hemoglobin (HbF). However, by 6 months of age, as the percentage of HbF decreases and the percentage of HbS increases approximately 6% of HbSS infants are symptomatic. This increases to 32% by age 1 year, 61% by age 2 years, and 96% by age 8 years [7]. Notable sequelae in children include: dactylitis, splenic sequestration, osteonecrosis/avascular necrosis, priapism, stroke, acute chest syndrome, and acute vasoocclusive pain crisis. Pulmonary arterial hypertension, myocardial infarction, sickle cell nephropathy, and proliferative retinopathy are SCD sequelae generally seen in adults. Although these manifestations are less likely to present in children, pediatricians should still maintain a high index of suspicion.

New approaches to management are needed to improve quality of life and long-term outcomes in patients with SCD. We summarize the newest advances in SCD with a focus on preventive care, including vaccinations and screening for disease complications, stroke prevention, and the newest medications and therapies on the horizon.

PREVENTIVE CARE AND SCREENING

Infection prevention

Infants with SCD are considered functionally asplenic for the purposes of infection prophylaxis and prevention. This places them at increased risk for serious infections from encapsulated organisms including *Haemophilus influenzae* type B, *Streptococcus pneumoniae*, and *Neisseria meningitidis*. Children with SCD require additional immunizations for protection against these organisms [8]. In 2014, the Centers for Disease Control and Prevention began recommending the MCV4 vaccine Menveo for infants with SCD greater than or equal to 2 months of age. In addition to the standard immunization schedule, which includes a complete *H influenzae* type B and PCV13 series, patients with SCD require additional vaccines (Table 1) [8,9]. As further protection against infection it is also recommended that patients with HbSS receive penicillin prophylaxis per the National Heart, Lung and Blood Institute (NHLBI) 2014 recommendations (Table 2) [10]. Parents should also be educated to seek medical attention if fever occurs. Children with SCD should have a medical home with a pediatrician who is familiar with these recommendations to ensure appropriate preventative care.

Pulmonary hypertension screening

Although adults with SCD and pulmonary hypertension (PH) are at increased risk of morbidity and mortality [11,12], currently there are conflicting guidelines for PH in children with SCD. PH occurs in 10.5% of adults with SCD [13]. Half of the patients with PH have left ventricular dysfunction, and the other half have precapillary hypertension as a result of vasculopathy secondary to intravascular hemolysis, chronic thromboembolism, or chronic upregulated hypoxic responses to anemia, hypoxemia, or microvascular obstruction [14].

Elevated tricuspid regurgitant jet velocity (TRV) on echocardiography is used as a screening method for PH. Consensus guidelines for PH in adults with SCD, published by the American Thoracic Society, the American College of Chest Physicians, and the Pulmonary Hypertension Association, recommend screening every 1 to 3 years with echocardiogram or by measuring plasma N-terminal pro–B-type natriuretic peptide to identify patients at high risk for morbidity and mortality [15]. Per these guidelines, a screening TRV greater than 3 m/s prompts right heart catheterization. A TRV between 2.5 and 3 m/s prompts further stratification. A TRV greater than 2.5 m/s and an elevated N-terminal pro–B-type natriuretic peptide (>164 pg/mL) or a decreased 6-minute walk distance (<333 m) have a positive predictive value of 62% for PH [16].

The evidence in children is less clear. In two separate studies, children with SCD had a baseline TRV greater than 2.5 m/s with a prevalence of 19% to 33%, indicating that TRV is a poor independent predictor of morbidity in children [17,18]. In one study [17], mean TRV in the study population improved without intervention. The risk of death is generally low in children, and there have been no sufficiently long longitudinal studies to show mortality risk [11]. The 2015 guidelines from the American Thoracic Society on Pediatric Pulmonary Hypertension are summarized in Table 3 [19]. Until further evidence is available, physicians caring for children with SCD who have cardiopulmonary symptoms must maintain a low threshold for PH evaluation. The timing of screening for PH in children younger than 8 years remains at the discretion of the physician.

Renal disease screening

Sickle cell nephropathy is a major cause of morbidity and mortality in patients with SCD. Renal disease ranges from glomerulopathy to tubular defects, and

Table 1
Vaccinations

Vaccination		Dosing schedule	Considerations
PPSV23 (Pneumovax)		First dose at ≥2 y of age with a booster vaccine 5 y after the first dose	Should be given ≥8 wk after completion of PCV13 series
Meningococcal vaccines			
MCV4	Menactra	First dose at ≥2 y of age Given as 2 doses 2 mo apart If primary series is completed when child is <7 y of age give initial booster after 3 y, then every 5 y thereafter	Approved for children ≥2 y of age Should be given at least 4 wk after completion of the PCV13 series
	Menvo	Children 2–18 mo: 4 doses at 2, 4, 6, and 12 mo Children 19–23 mo who have had no prior doses: 2 doses 3 mo apart Children >2 y who have had no prior doses: 2 doses 2 mo apart If primary series is completed when child is <7 y of age give initial booster after 3 y, then every 5 y thereafter	Approved for children ≥2 mo of age
MenB	Trumenba	3 doses given 0, 1–2, and 6 mo apart	Approved for children ≥10 y of age
	Bexsero	2 doses given at least 1 mo apart	Approved for children ≥10 y of age

Table 2
Penicillin prophylaxis: recommendations from the NHLBI 2014 expert panel report

Recommendation	Quality of evidence
HbSS patients: oral penicillin twice daily until 5 y old 125 mg for age <3 y 250 mg for age ≥3 y	Strong recommendation, moderate-quality evidence
Discontinue penicillin prophylaxis at 5 y old unless they have had splenectomy or invasive pneumococcal infection	Weak recommendation, moderate-quality evidence
HbSC and HbSB + thalassemia patients: consider withholding penicillin prophylaxis unless they have had splenectomy	Weak recommendation, low-quality evidence

Adapted from National Heart Lung and Blood Institute. Sickle Cell Disease. Available at: https://www.nhlbi.nih.gov/health-topics/sickle-cell-disease. Accessed September 2019.

often results in end-stage renal disease [20,21]. Although the exact pathophysiologic mechanism is unknown and likely multifactorial, it is likely that sickle cell nephropathy is mostly secondary to functional vasculopathy, with a combination of medullary hypoperfusion and cortical hyperperfusion [20,22]. Albuminuria is the most common manifestation of renal disease in SCD [20,22]. Persistent excretion of albumin between 30 and 300 mg/d is considered

Table 3
2015 guidelines from the American Thoracic Society on pediatric pulmonary hypertension

Recommendation	Level of evidence
Early screening with Doppler echocardiogram is reasonable for children with hemolytic hemoglobinopathies who develop cardiorespiratory symptoms.	Class IIa; level of evidence C
It is reasonable for children with SCD to undergo screening by 8 y of age or earlier in patients with frequent cardiorespiratory symptoms.	Class I; level of evidence B
Children with SCD who have evidence of PH by echocardiogram should have further testing with polysomnography, pulmonary function testing, evaluation for thromboembolic disease, and assessment for oxygenation.	Class I; level of evidence C
Children with SCD should undergo cardiac catheterization before initiation of treatment of PH.	Class I; level of evidence C

Adapted from Abman SH, Hansmann G, Archer SL, et al. Pediatric pulmonary hypertension: Guidelines From the American Heart Association and American Thoracic Society. Circulation 2015;132(21):2037-2099.

microalbuminuria, whereas albumin excretion higher than 300 mg/d is considered macroalbuminuria [21]. In a large prospective study, the median age for onset of "sickle renal failure" was 23.1 years and proteinuria was a strong predictor of renal failure [23]. Multiple studies report an 18% to 30% prevalence of microalbuminuria in children with SCD [24–27].

The most recent consensus screening recommendations for renal disease in children with SCD, from the NHLBI in 2014, recommend screening individuals with SCD for proteinuria beginning at age 10. Repeat screening should be performed annually if the result is negative. For positive results, a first morning void urine albumin/creatinine ratio should be performed and if abnormal consultation or referral to a renal specialist should be made [28].

In addition to microalbuminuria, other biomarkers for sickle cell nephropathy have been identified, although not yet validated, including hyperuricemia [29]. Hyperfiltration, which is measured by cystatin C levels, has been associated with development of sickle cell nephropathy [27,30]. Prospective studies are needed to evaluate progression of renal disease in children with SCD and appropriate screening methods.

Stroke and neurocognitive screening

The neurologic complications of sickle cell during childhood range from overt strokes that are often associated with a moyamoya-like vasculopathy to subtle neurocognitive changes affecting cognitive processing, executive function, and mood. Overt stroke seems to affect children with SCA, tending to spare children with other genotypes, such as sickle cell SC. Roughly 11% of SCA patients suffer an overt stroke during childhood with the risk being greatest from 2 to 10 years of age. Stroke in children is primarily ischemic; hemorrhagic stroke may occur but tends to be more prevalent in adults [31].

All patients and parents of children with SCD must be aware of this potential complication and understand that signs of stroke require emergent medical care. Stroke should be suspected in a child with SCD presenting with acute neurologic symptoms that can include headache, seizure, or focal neurologic deficits. If stroke is suspected, emergent neurologic consultation should be obtained and computed tomography of the head followed by MRI. Magnetic resonance angiography, if available, should also be performed. If the patient is found to have had a stroke, an exchange transfusion should be initiated promptly [32].

The most valid test for predicting the risk of stroke is the transcranial Doppler ultrasound (TCD), which is recommended for screening children with SCD for stroke. TCD measures the flow of blood through the proximal portion of the middle cerebral artery and terminal portion of the internal carotid artery. Faster flow indicates stenosis in the affected artery and a higher risk of stroke [33]. Based on this observation, the National Institutes of Health (NIH) funded the STOP trial, which tested the use of TCD as a screening tool in children with SCA who were undergoing chronic blood transfusion therapy. This trial ended early because patients treated with transfusions had less than

1% risk of stroke per year compared with 10% in the control group, an overall 92% reduction in stroke risk [34]. The follow-up STOP 2 trial attempted to determine if stopping transfusions after at least 30 months was feasible. Unfortunately, it was stopped early after a significant number of patients reverted back to elevated TCD scores or suffered strokes after transfusions were stopped [35]. Based on the STOP trials, the NHLBI recommends that all children with SCA receive once yearly TCD screening using the STOP trial technique [10].

Although the STOP, STOP2, and TWiTCH (discussed later) trials used nonimaging TCD, many institutions use imaging TCD to evaluate stroke risk. There has been much debate about cutoff values between imaging TCD and traditional TCD, which would impact the timing of transfusion therapy initiation [36–38]. The new American Society of Hematology guidelines on SCD-related cerebrovascular disease, expected in 2020, will likely include the role of hydroxyurea for primary prophylaxis of stroke and provide guidance for using imaging TCD screening for primary prophylaxis. How can this be updated?

The risk of a second stroke following an initial stroke in SCA is roughly 50% in the first 2 years and 66% in the subsequent 9 years [39]. Therefore, children should be started on a chronic blood transfusion regimen to keep HbS percent less than 30% and with iron chelation to decrease the chance of a second stroke. Despite regular blood transfusions, almost half of children with a prior stroke have progressive cerebral events including silent infarcts and overt strokes [40].

A much larger percentage of patients with SCD suffer more subtle neurocognitive complications because of silent strokes. MRI imaging in the BABY HUG trial (discussed later) revealed that 30% to 40% of children with SCA had had silent strokes and 13% of infants with SCA had had silent stroke by a mean age of 14 months. To date, there have been no randomized controlled trials on the primary prevention of silent stroke in SCD. SIT, a randomized controlled trial for the secondary prevention of silent stroke, included 196 children with no history of overt stroke but with one or more silent strokes. They were randomized to either receive chronic blood transfusions or observation only; hydroxyurea was not allowed. The incidence of a stroke or silent stroke in the transfused versus observed group was 2.0 and 4.8 events, respectively, per 100 years at risk showing that transfusion therapy significantly reduced the risk of recurrent infarcts [41]. The authors concluded that all children with SCA should undergo an MRI of the brain during early school age for assessment of silent stroke. If a past silent stroke is found, chronic blood transfusions should be started for secondary prevention of silent stroke and formal testing should be implemented to assess for neurocognitive dysfunction.

Numerous studies have demonstrated a decline in neurocognitive function in children and adults with SCD regardless of overt or silent stroke occurrence. A meta-analysis of 110 studies of SCD showed significant deficits across all neurocognitive domains, age groups, and infarct status. Defects in full scale IQ, verbal reasoning, perceptual reasoning, and executive function increased from preschool to school age, with deficits smaller in adults versus children, likely because of sampling bias in adult studies. Deficits in all domains increased from no infarct/stroke to silent stroke to overt stroke [42]. A systematic review showed that children with SCD and no apparent MRI abnormality have significantly lower IQ than healthy control subjects (7 points). SCD patients with prior stroke had the lowest IQ followed by those with prior silent stroke and those with no prior history of MRI abnormalities [43]. These results indicate that physicians should screen all children with SCD for neurocognitive deficits. If present, formal neurocognitive testing should be performed and additional services or accommodations may need to be implemented at the child's school.

MEDICAL MANAGEMENT

Hydroxyurea

Hydroxyurea was the first Food and Drug Administration (FDA)-approved medication for the treatment of SCD. It increases the production of HbF, reducing the amount of HbS, thereby decreasing sickling and vasoocclusion. A landmark study in pediatric SCD patients was the 2011 BABY HUG trial, in which 193 infants with either HbSS or HbSß^0 thalassemia were randomized to receive hydroxyurea or placebo. The treated patients had a significant decrease in pain, acute chest syndrome, dactylitis, hospitalization, and transfusion. Side effects were minimal with the most common being mild-moderate neutropenia (absolute neutrophil count [ANC] 500–1250). Severe neutropenia (ANC <500) was rare (5%) [44]. Based on these results the NHLBI 2014 expert panel recommends that hydroxyurea should be offered to all children 9 months of age and older with SCD regardless of their clinical severity [10]. Hydroxyurea gained FDA approval in 2017 after the results of the European Sickle Cell Disease Cohort (ESCORT-HU) supported the results of the BABY HUG trial showing improved symptoms of SCD with few side effects [45]. The efficacy of hydroxyurea to decrease pain crises and acute complications was confirmed in a 2017 Cochrane review [46]. Unfortunately, the effects of hydroxyurea on chronic complications and its long-term effects remain unknown, which is being addressed in several observational cohorts [45,47].

The use of hydroxyurea for stroke prevention was the focus of the landmark TWiTCH and SWiTCH trials. Chronic transfusion therapy is effective for primary stroke prevention but is expensive; time consuming for patients; and has side effects, such as transfusion reactions, alloimmunization, and chronic iron overload leading to organ failure. The TWiTCH trial evaluated whether hydroxyurea could be substituted for chronic blood transfusions. This NIH-funded trial enrolled children who were at increased risk for stroke based on the STOP criteria without a history of severe vasculopathy or history of silent stroke by MRI and magnetic resonance angiography. After a year of chronic transfusion therapy, patients transitioned to hydroxyurea therapy. TCD velocity, the primary end point, was used as a surrogate for stroke risk. The hydroxyurea arm was equivalent with no difference in TCD velocity or progression of vasculopathy or stroke compared with chronic transfusion

[48]. Transition to hydroxyurea is considered as an alternative to chronic transfusion therapy following thorough discussion with the patient and family outlining the risks, benefits, and limitations of current knowledge regarding optimal therapy.

Hydroxyurea for secondary prevention of stroke was investigated in the NIH-funded SWiTCH trial. Patients were transitioned to hydroxyurea from chronic blood transfusions, but the study closed early because of an increased number of neurologic events in the hydroxyurea group. There was futility in reaching the primary end point of decreasing iron overload in the hydroxyurea group. The authors concluded that chronic exchange transfusion is the most effective therapy for the secondary prevention of stroke [49]. Several observational studies have suggested a reduction in secondary strokes using hydroxyurea only, so when blood transfusion therapy is not feasible, hydroxyurea versus no therapy is preferred [50].

To date there are no randomized controlled trials to determine if hydroxyurea is effective in preventing silent strokes. We conducted a systematic review of hydroxyurea for silent stroke prevention and found a trend toward benefit with hydroxyurea, although more evidence is needed to confirm this finding [51].

L-Glutamine

L-Glutamine (Endari) is the first FDA-approved treatment of SCD since the introduction of hydroxyurea. L-Glutamine gained approval based on the results of a phase 3 multicenter randomized, placebo-controlled, double-blind clinical trial. It was hypothesized that administration of L-glutamine would reduce oxidative stress and thus decrease the number of pain crises in patients with SCD. Niihara and colleagues [52] demonstrated a statistically significant decrease in pain crises and hospitalizations among treated patients versus placebo. This study, however, is controversial because of high dropout rates. There are also concerns that cost and adherence will be barriers to routine use.

Crizanlizumab-tmca

The pathophysiology of vasoocclusive crises in SCD is complex. Abnormalities in blood flow, which can ultimately contribute to vascular obstruction, ischemia, and pain, are in part secondary to adhesion of leukocytes and sickled erythrocytes to the endothelium during inflammation [53,54]. P-selectin, an important adhesion molecule found in endothelial cells, is expressed during inflammation resulting in adhesion of leukocytes and sickle erythrocytes to the vessel surface [55]. It was thus hypothesized that blocking P-selectin in SCD could decrease vasoocclusion and pain crises.

Crizanlizumab-tmca was developed as a monoclonal antibody that binds and blocks P-selectin. The SUSTAIN trial assessed the efficacy and safety of crizanlizumab-tmca in patients with SCD [53,56]. There was a 45.3% lower median pain crisis rate per year in the high-dose crizanlizumab-tmca versus placebo group ($P = .01$) [53]. The investigators concluded that crizanlizumab-tmca is effective in decreasing pain crises, leading to FDA approval in

November 2019 for its use in SCD patients greater than or equal to 16 years of age. An ongoing phase II multicenter study is assessing appropriate dosing and evaluating safety of crizanlizumab-tmca in the pediatric population [57].

Voxelotor

Additionally, such agents as voxelotor are being evaluated for their ability to change hemoglobin structure to prevent sickling. Voxelotor targets hemoglobin causing structural changes that increase the oxygen affinity; it is thought that this increased oxygen affinity will prevent HbS polymerization and sickling [58,59]. In a phase I/II study of voxelotor, Howard and colleagues [60] treated SCD patients with voxelotor and demonstrated a median hemoglobin increase of 1.0 g/dL, improved laboratory markers of hemolysis, and a greater than 70% reduction in sickled red cells. The HOPE Trial compared the safety and efficacy of two different doses of voxelotor. At 24 weeks of treatment the percentages of SCD patients with a greater than 1.0 g/dL increase in hemoglobin were 59%, 38%, and 9% in the 1500-mg voxelotor, 900-mg voxelotor, and the placebo group, respectively [61]. However, the incidence of vasoocclusive crises did not differ significantly between groups [61]. Based on the results of this trial voxelotor has also gained FDA approval, as of November 2019, for SCD patients 12 years of age and older.

Ongoing clinical studies of voxelotor in the pediatric population include the HOPE-KIDS1 Trial, which is investigating its safety and efficacy in patients 12 to 17 years of age, and NCT02850406, which is investigating its effects on TCD velocity in patients ages 4 to 17 years [62]. Although early results of voxelotor as a disease-modifying agent are promising there are still many unanswered questions, particularly its effects on clinical outcomes.

BONE MARROW TRANSPLANT

Currently the only curative therapy for SCD is hematopoietic stem cell transplantation (HSCT). Johnson and colleagues reported the first case of a child with SCD receiving HSCT in the *New England Journal of Medicine* in 1984. The 8-year-old girl who had developed acute myeloid leukemia received an HSCT from a matched sibling donor with sickle cell trait. Seven months after transplant she had stable levels of hemoglobin A and hemoglobin S consistent with sickle-cell trait; she remains alive several decades later [63,64]. Transplant is generally reserved for patients who continue to have significant disease complications (eg, frequent pain crises, acute chest syndrome, stroke, elevated TCD) [65–69]. Considerations for use of HSCT for SCD include the optimal age and timing of transplant, donor type, and conditioning regimen.

Several studies have investigated the impact of age at time of transplant on overall outcomes and survival. A large retrospective cohort study by Gluckman and colleagues [70] assessed 1000 patients who received an HLA-identical sibling transplant for SCD. The 5-year overall survival of patients transplanted at less than 16 versus greater than or equal to 16 years of age was 95% versus 81%, respectively ($P<.001$). Rates of acute and chronic graft-versus-host disease were also higher with increasing age [70]. Arnold and colleagues [71] also showed that children transplanted at greater than or equal to 10 years of age had increased mortality (hazard ratio, 21.21; $P \leq .05$). Although children transplanted at a younger age have improved outcomes they often have not developed the severe comorbidities seen in older SCD patients. Decisions regarding transplant in young children are difficult because the potential for morbidity and mortality associated with transplant must be weighed against the potential morbidity and mortality associated with disease. Additionally, there are no prognostic models for predicting which SCD patients will have a more severe course, making it difficult to weigh these risks and benefits in young, asymptomatic children.

A significant barrier to HSCT in SCD patients is availability of a suitable donor. The preferred donor is an HLA-matched sibling without SCD, although sickle cell trait is acceptable. Alternative donors, including mismatched (haploidentical) related donors and matched unrelated donors, are being investigated in clinical trials, but these donors are not widely available and using them for transplant is currently considered experimental. The type of conditioning regimen, which includes the combination of medications and/or radiation used to eradicate the host marrow in preparation for transplant, must also be considered. Myeloablative regimens are used to treat malignancies and fully eradicate the cancer cells. These regimens, however, can cause significant organ toxicity and even infertility. Thus, current clinical trials are investigating the efficacy and outcomes with reduced-intensity regimens for transplants in the SCD population.

Although HSCT may provide opportunities for cure, further studies are needed to determine the safety and efficacy of donor types and conditioning regimens, and longitudinal studies are needed to assess outcomes.

GENE THERAPY

In addition to HSCT, gene therapy is being explored as a curative option for SCD. The ultimate goal of gene therapy is to replace a patient's abnormal gene with new genetic material. Through a process similar to a bone marrow transplant the patient's bone marrow is eradicated and then replaced with their own genetically modified stem cells [72]. Ongoing clinical trials are investigating the use of gene therapy technology to increase HbF production or modify the beta-globin gene to inhibit HbS polymerization [72,73].

The first case of an SCD patient treated with gene therapy was published in the *New England Journal of Medicine* in 2017. The boy was 13 years old and failed to show significant improvement on hydroxyurea, thus was started on chronic transfusions. He had multiple episodes of vasoocclusive crises, acute chest syndrome, bilateral hip osteonecrosis, and had undergone cholecystectomy and splenectomy. As part of the clinical trial he underwent autologous transplant after gene modification with a lentiviral vector encoding a human beta-globin variant that inhibits HbS polymerization. He showed significant clinical improvement without sickle cell–related complications or hospitalizations after 15 months from transplant and was able to discontinue all medications including pain medications [74]. Gene therapy offers a potential cure for SCD without the need for a bone marrow donor or the toxicity associated with traditional conditioning regimens for HSCT. More data, however, are needed on the safety, efficacy, and long-term outcomes of this new therapy.

SUMMARY

- Increased awareness of the chronic complications of SCD has led to improvement in screening protocols and better preventive care
- Multiple medications, and an increased role for chronic blood transfusions, are now available for SCD for prevention and treatment of its complications
- New therapies focus on curing the disease through HSCT and gene therapy

Disclosure

The authors have nothing to disclose.

References

[1] Dueker ND, Della-Morte D, Rundek T, et al. Sickle cell trait and renal function in Hispanics in the United States: the Northern Manhattan study. Ethn Dis 2017;27(1):11–4.
[2] National Center on Birth Defects and Developmental Disabilities Center for Disease Control and Prevention. Sickle Cell Disease (SCD) Data and Statistics. 2019. Available at: https://www.cdc.gov/ncbddd/sicklecell/data.html. Accessed September 25, 2019.
[3] Macharia AW, Mochamah G, Uyoga S, et al. The clinical epidemiology of sickle cell anemia In Africa. Am J Hematol 2018;93(3):363–70.
[4] Weatherall D, Hofman K, Rodgers G, et al. A case for developing north-south partnerships for research in sickle cell disease. Blood 2005;105(3):921–3.
[5] Browning JA, Staines HM, Robinson HC, et al. The effect of deoxygenation on whole-cell conductance of red blood cells from healthy individuals and patients with sickle cell disease. Blood 2007;109(6):2622–9.
[6] US Preventive Service Task Force. Screening for sickle cell disease in newborns: recommendation statement. Am Fam Physician 2008;77(9):1300–2.
[7] Bainbridge R, Higgs DR, Maude GH, et al. Clinical presentation of homozygous sickle cell disease. J Pediatr 1985;106(6):881–5.
[8] American Academy of Pediatrics. Active and passive immunization. Immunization in special clinical circumstances: asplenia and functional asplenia. In: Kimberlin DW, Brady MT, Jackson MA, et al, editors. Red book: 2018 report of the committee on infectious diseases. 31st edition. Itasca (IL): American Academy of Pediatrics; 2018. p. 88–90.
[9] Robinson CL, Bernstein H, Romero JR, et al. Advisory Committee on Immunization Practices recommended immunization schedules for children and adolescents aged 18 years or younger - United States, 2019. MMWR Morb Mortal Wkly Rep 2019;68(5):112–4.
[10] National Heart Lung and Blood Institute. Sickle Cell Disease. Available at: https://www.nhlbi.nih.gov/health-topics/sickle-cell-disease. Accessed September 25, 2019.
[11] Willen SM, Gladwin MT. What is the role of screening for pulmonary hypertension in adults and children with sickle cell disease? Hematology 2017;2017(1):431–4.
[12] Castro O. Pulmonary hypertension in sickle cell disease: cardiac catheterization results and survival. Blood 2003;101(4):1257–61.
[13] Mehari A, Alam S, Tian X, et al. Hemodynamic predictors of mortality in adults with sickle cell disease. Am J Respir Crit Care Med 2013;187(8):840–7.
[14] Gordeuk VR, Castro OL, Machado RF. Pathophysiology and treatment of pulmonary hypertension in sickle cell disease. Blood 2016;127(7):820–8.

[15] Klings ES, Machado RF, Barst RJ, et al. An official American Thoracic Society clinical practice guideline: diagnosis, risk stratification, and management of pulmonary hypertension of sickle cell disease. Am J Respir Crit Care Med 2014;189(6):727–40.
[16] Parent F, Bachir D, Inamo J, et al. A hemodynamic study of pulmonary hypertension in sickle cell disease. N Engl J Med 2011;365(1):44–53.
[17] Hebson C, New T, Record E, et al. Elevated tricuspid regurgitant velocity as a marker for pulmonary hypertension in children with sickle cell disease. J Pediatr Hematol Oncol 2015;37(2):134–9.
[18] Liem RI, Nevin MA, Prestridge A, et al. Tricuspid regurgitant jet velocity elevation and its relationship to lung function in pediatric sickle cell disease. Pediatr Pulmonol 2009;44(3):281–9.
[19] Abman SH, Hansmann G, Archer SL, et al. Pediatric pulmonary hypertension: guidelines From the American Heart Association and American Thoracic Society. Circulation 2015;132(21):2037–99.
[20] Hariri E, Mansour A, El Alam A, et al. Sickle cell nephropathy: an update on pathophysiology, diagnosis, and treatment. Int Urol Nephrol 2018;50(6):1075–83.
[21] Ataga KI, Derebail VK, Archer DR. The glomerulopathy of sickle cell disease. Am J Hematol 2014;89(9):907–14.
[22] Nath KA, Hebbel RP. Sickle cell disease: renal manifestations and mechanisms. Nat Rev Nephrol 2015;11(3):161–71.
[23] Powars DR. Chronic renal failure in sickle cell disease: risk factors, clinical course, and mortality. Ann Intern Med 1991;115(8):614.
[24] Datta V, Ayengar JR, Karpate S, et al. Microalbuminuria as a predictor of early glomerular injury in children with sickle cell disease. Indian J Pediatr 2003;70(4):307–9.
[25] McKie KT, Hanevold CD, Hernandez C, et al. Prevalence, prevention, and treatment of microalbuminuria and proteinuria in children with sickle cell disease. J Pediatr Hematol Oncol 2007;29(3):140–4.
[26] Dharnidharka VR, Dabbagh S, Atiyeh B, et al. Prevalence of microalbuminuria in children with sickle cell disease. Pediatr Nephrol 1998;12(6):475–8.
[27] Aygun B, Mortier NA, Smeltzer MP, et al. Glomerular hyperfiltration and albuminuria in children with sickle cell anemia. Pediatr Nephrol 2011;26(8):1285–90.
[28] National Heart, Lung, and Blood Institute. Evidence-based management of sickle cell disease: expert panel report, 2014. Bethesda (MD): National Heart, Lung, and Blood Institute, US Department of Health and Human Services; 2014. Available at: https://www.nhlbi.nih.gov/sites/default/files/media/docs/sickle-cell-disease-report%20020816_0.pdf. Accessed September 2019.
[29] Lebensburger JD, Cutter GR, Howard TH, et al. Evaluating risk factors for chronic kidney disease in pediatric patients with sickle cell anemia. Pediatr Nephrol 2017;32(9):1565–73.
[30] Lebensburger JD, Aban I, Pernell B, et al. Hyperfiltration during early childhood precedes albuminuria in pediatric sickle cell nephropathy. Am J Hematol 2019;94(4):417–23.
[31] Ohene-Frempong K, Weiner SJ, Sleeper LA, et al. Cerebrovascular accidents in sickle cell disease: rates and risk factors. Blood 1998;91(1):288–94.
[32] Yawn BP, Buchanan GR, Afenyi-Annan AN, et al. Management of sickle cell disease: summary of the 2014 evidence-based report by expert panel members. JAMA 2014;312(10):1033–48.
[33] Adams RJ, McKie VC, Carl EM, et al. Long-term stroke risk in children with sickle cell disease screened with transcranial Doppler. Ann Neurol 1997;42(5):699–704.
[34] Adams RJ. Prevention of stroke in sickle cell anemia. J Law Med Ethics 2014;42(2):135–8.
[35] Adams RJ, Brambilla D, Optimizing Primary Stroke Prevention in Sickle Cell Anemia (STOP 2) Trial Investigators. Discontinuing prophylactic transfusions used to prevent stroke in sickle cell disease. N Engl J Med 2005;353(26):2769–78.

[36] Jones AM, Seibert JJ, Nichols FT, et al. Comparison of transcranial color Doppler imaging (TCDI) and transcranial Doppler (TCD) in children with sickle-cell anemia. Pediatr Radiol 2001;31(7):461–9.
[37] Padayachee ST, Thomas N, Arnold AJ, et al. Problems with implementing a standardised transcranial Doppler screening programme: impact of instrumentation variation on STOP classification. Pediatr Radiol 2012;42(4):470–4.
[38] Mazzucco S, Diomedi M, Qureshi A, et al. Transcranial Doppler screening for stroke risk in children with sickle cell disease: a systematic review. Int J Stroke 2017;12(6):580–8.
[39] Powars D, Wilson B, Imbus C, et al. The natural history of stroke in sickle cell disease. Am J Med 1978;65(3):461–71.
[40] Hulbert ML, McKinstry RC, Lacey JL, et al. Silent cerebral infarcts occur despite regular blood transfusion therapy after first strokes in children with sickle cell disease. Blood 2011;117(3): 772–9.
[41] DeBaun MR, Gordon M, McKinstry RC, et al. Controlled trial of transfusions for silent cerebral infarcts in sickle cell anemia. N Engl J Med 2014;371(8):699–710.
[42] Prussien KV, Jordan LC, DeBaun MR, et al. Cognitive function in sickle cell disease across domains, cerebral infarct status, and the lifespan: a meta-analysis. J Pediatr Psychol 2019;4(8):948–58.
[43] Kawadler JM, Clayden JD, Clark CA, et al. Intelligence quotient in paediatric sickle cell disease: a systematic review and meta-analysis. Dev Med Child Neurol 2016;58(7):672–9.
[44] Wang WC, Ware RE, Miller ST, et al. Hydroxycarbamide in very young children with sickle-cell anaemia: a multicentre, randomised, controlled trial (BABY HUG). Lancet 2011;377(9778):1663–72.
[45] de Montalembert M, Oevermann L, Benkerrou M, et al. ESCORT-HU paediatric, real-life experience of using hydroxycarbamide to treat children affected with sickle cell disease: the ESCORT-HU Cohort Study. Lancet. 2019. Available at: https://papers.ssrn.com/sol3/papers.cfm?abstract_id=3414425. Accessed October 14, 2019.
[46] Nevitt SJ, Jones AP, Howard J. Hydroxyurea (hydroxycarbamide) for sickle cell disease. Cochrane Database Syst Rev 2017;4:CD002202.
[47] Long term effects of hydroxyurea therapy in children with sickle cell disease. Available at: https://clinicaltrials.gov/ct2/show/NCT00305175?term=NCT00305175&draw=2&rank=1. ClinicalTrials.gov identifier: NCT00305175. Accessed October 14, 2019.
[48] Ware RE, Davis BR, Schultz WH, et al. Hydroxycarbamide versus chronic transfusion for maintenance of transcranial Doppler flow velocities in children with sickle cell anaemia. TCD With Transfusions Changing to Hydroxyurea (TWiTCH): a multicentre, open-label, phase 3, non-inferiority trial. Lancet 2016;387(10019):661–70.
[49] Ware RE, Helms RW, Investigators SW. Stroke With Transfusions Changing to Hydroxyurea (SWiTCH). Blood 2012;119(17):3925–32.
[50] Kassim AA, Galadanci NA, Pruthi S, et al. How I treat and manage strokes in sickle cell disease. Blood 2015;125(22):3401–10.
[51] Hasson C, Veling L, Rico J, et al. The role of hydroxyurea to prevent silent stroke in sickle cell disease: systematic review and meta-analysis. Medicine (Baltimore) 2019;98(51): e18225.
[52] Niihara Y, Smith WR, Stark CW. A phase 3 trial of L-glutamine in sickle cell disease. N Engl J Med 2018;379(19):1880.
[53] Ataga KI, Kutlar A, Kanter J, et al. Crizanlizumab for the prevention of pain crises in sickle cell disease. N Engl J Med 2017;376(5):429–39.
[54] Kutlar A, Ataga KI, McMahon L, et al. A potent oral P-selectin blocking agent improves microcirculatory blood flow and a marker of endothelial cell injury in patients with sickle cell disease. Am J Hematol 2012;87(5):536–9.
[55] Matsui NM, Borsig L, Rosen SD, et al. P-selectin mediates the adhesion of sickle erythrocytes to the endothelium. Blood 2001;98(6):1955–62.

[56] Kutlar A, Kanter J, Liles DK, et al. Effect of crizanlizumab on pain crises in subgroups of patients with sickle cell disease: a SUSTAIN study analysis. Am J Hematol 2019;94(1):55–61.
[57] Study of dose confirmation and safety of crizanlizumab in pediatric sickle cell disease patients. Available at: https://clinicaltrials.gov/ct2/show/NCT03474965?term=NCT03474965&draw=2&rank=1. ClinicalTrials.gov identifier: NCT03474965. Accessed October 14, 2019.
[58] Metcalf B, Chuang C, Dufu K, et al. Discovery of GBT440, an orally bioavailable R-state stabilizer of sickle cell hemoglobin. ACS Med Chem Lett 2017;8(3):321–6.
[59] Oksenberg D, Dufu K, Patel MP, et al. GBT440 increases haemoglobin oxygen affinity, reduces sickling and prolongs RBC half-life in a murine model of sickle cell disease. Br J Haematol 2016;175(1):141–53.
[60] Howard J, Hemmaway CJ, Telfer P, et al. A phase 1/2 ascending dose study and open-label extension study of voxelotor in patients with sickle cell disease. Blood 2019;133(17):1865–75.
[61] Vichinsky E, Hoppe CC, Ataga KI, et al. A phase 3 randomized trial of voxelotor in sickle cell disease. N Engl J Med 2019;381(6):509–19.
[62] Study to evaluate the effect of GBT440 in pediatrics with sickle cell disease. Available at: https://clinicaltrials.gov/ct2/show/NCT02850406?term=NCT02850406&draw=2&rank=1. ClinicalTrials.gov identifier: NCT02850406. Accessed October 15, 2019.
[63] Johnson FL, Look AT, Gockerman J, et al. Bone-marrow transplantation in a patient with sickle-cell anemia. N Engl J Med 1984;311(12):780–3.
[64] Fitzhugh CD, Abraham AA, Tisdale JF, et al. Hematopoietic stem cell transplantation for patients with sickle cell disease: progress and future directions. Hematol Oncol Clin North Am 2014;28(6):1171–85.
[65] Alfraih F, Aljurf M, Fitzhugh CD, et al. Alternative donor allogeneic hematopoietic cell transplantation for hemoglobinopathies. Semin Hematol 2016;53(2):120–8.
[66] Kassim AA, Sharma D. Hematopoietic stem cell transplantation for sickle cell disease: the changing landscape. Hematol Oncol Stem Cell Ther 2017;10(4):259–66.
[67] Bernaudin F, Pondarre C, Glambrun C, et al. Allogeneic/matched related transplantation for B-thalassemia and sickle cell anemia. In: Malik P, Tisdale J, editors. Gene and cell therapies for beta-globinopathies (Advances in Experimental Medicine and Biology, American Society of Gene & Cell Therapy, vol. 1013. New York: Springer; 2017. p. P89–122.
[68] Bernaudin F. Why, who, when, and how? Rationale for considering allogeneic stem cell transplantation in children with sickle cell disease. J Clin Med 2019;8(10):1523.
[69] Bernaudin F, Verlhac S, Peffault de Latour R, et al. Association of matched sibling donor hematopoietic stem cell transplantation with transcranial Doppler velocities in children with sickle cell anemia. JAMA 2019;321(3):266–76.
[70] Gluckman E, Cappelli B, Bernaudin F, et al. Sickle cell disease: an international survey of results of HLA-identical sibling hematopoietic stem cell transplantation. Blood 2017;129(11):1548–56.
[71] Arnold SD, Brazauskas R, He N, et al. Clinical risks and healthcare utilization of hematopoietic cell transplantation for sickle cell disease in the USA using merged databases. Haematologica 2017;102(11):1823–32.
[72] Gene transfer for sickle cell disease. Available at: https://clinicaltrials.gov/ct2/show/NCT03282656?term=NCT03282656&draw=2&rank=1. ClinicalTrials.gov identifier: NCT03282656. Accessed October 21, 2019.
[73] Stem cell gene therapy for sickle cell disease. Available at: https://clinicaltrials.gov/ct2/show/NCT02247843?term=NCT02247843&draw=2&rank=1. ClinicalTrials.gov identifier: NCT02247843. Accessed October 21, 2019.
[74] Ribeil JA, Hacein-Bey-Abina S, Payen E, et al. Gene therapy in a patient with sickle cell disease. N Engl J Med 2017;376(9):848–55.

Advances in Pediatrics 67 (2020) 73–91

ADVANCES IN PEDIATRICS

Type 1 Diabetes in Youth and Technology-Based Advances in Management

Christopher Ferber, MD[a], Catherine S. Mao, MD[b,c], Jennifer K. Yee, MD[b,c,*]

[a]Department of Pediatrics, Harbor-UCLA Medical Center, 1000 West Carson Street, Harbor Box 446, Torrance, CA 90509, USA; [b]Division of Endocrinology, Department of Pediatrics, David Geffen School of Medicine at UCLA, Harbor-UCLA Medical Center, 1000 West Carson Street, Harbor Box 446, Torrance, CA 90509, USA; [c]The Lundquist Institute of Biomedical Innvoation at Harbor-UCLA, 1124 West Carson Street, Torrance, CA 90502, USA

Keywords

• Type 1 diabetes (T1D) • Insulin • Insulin pump
• Continuous glucose monitor (CGM) • Closed-loop system • Islet cell transplant

Key points

- Type 1 diabetes (T1D) is a worldwide condition with incidence rates that are increasing.
- Pathogenesis of T1D is the formation of autoantibodies that destroy pancreatic insulin-producing beta cells.
- Lifelong exogenous insulin is the predominant treatment modality, and it can be delivered using recombinant human insulin or its analogues in various regimens via syringe, pen, or pump.
- Continuous glucose monitoring has revolutionized outpatient T1D management and recent advances in closed-loop insulin pump systems to autonomously modify insulin administration.
- Research into prevention of T1D or curative measures such as islet cell transplant have shown some promise and are ongoing.

EPIDEMIOLOGY

Type 1 diabetes (T1D) is a global disease, affecting 1.1 million children and adolescents throughout the world [1]. For children and adolescents in the

*Corresponding author. 1000 West Carson Street, Harbor Box 446, Torrance, CA 90509.
E-mail address: jyee2@dhs.lacounty.gov

https://doi.org/10.1016/j.yapd.2020.04.002
0065-3101/20/

United States, the SEARCH for Diabetes in Youth (SEARCH) study was designed to estimate the overall incidence and prevalence among patients less than 20 years old and characterize the variation of impact in populations across the country [2]. Conducted from 2001 to 2009, the SEARCH study involved multiple locations, with sites in Ohio, Colorado, South Carolina, California, Washington state, and Hawaii, as well as American Indian reservations in New Mexico and Arizona. The results of this study revealed that the prevalence of diabetes of all types increased from 1.8 per 1000 in 2001 to 2.2 per 1000 patients in 2009, which approached 200,000 total cases. This increase in prevalence was consistent for patients of all ages, sexes, and racial/ethnic backgrounds. Furthermore, comparison of incidence rates from 2002 to 2003 and 2008 to 2009 identified an increase as well. This increase was noted among all racial/ethnic groups, but it was highest among non-Hispanic white people. Another finding of interest was that, despite the increase among all other age groups, prevalence of patients 0 to 4 years of age remained stable from 2001 to 2009. Overall, the SEARCH study provided valuable recognition that T1D is a disease that is progressively affecting more Americans each year.

T1D worldwide varies across countries and racial/ethnic populations. From 1990 to 1994, the Diabetes Mondiale (DiaMond) Project group reported stark differences in the incidence of T1D across different countries [3]. The lowest incidence rates were seen in China and Venezuela, only amounting to 0.1 per 100,000 cases annually. In contrast, the highest incidence rates identified were 36.8 and 36.5 per 100,000 in Sardinia and Finland, respectively. In addition, the other countries found to have the highest incidence rates included Norway, Sweden, the United Kingdom, Canada, Portugal and New Zealand. In most countries, incidence increased with increasing age, and was found to be highest in the groups aged 10 to 14 years.

Regarding age of onset, previous publications on the epidemiology have noted that, although the onset of T1D occurs primarily during childhood and adolescence, about one-quarter of patients are diagnosed as adults [4]. In addition, although onset of other types of diabetes may occur in the first 2 decades of life, approximately 85% of youth diagnosed with diabetes are ultimately classified as type 1. For this reason, T1D was historically referred to as juvenile diabetes. Regarding sex differences, epidemiologic data suggest that both male and female youth are diagnosed with T1D at similar rates; however, there may be an increase of diagnoses occurring as adults among men. One additional factor that may have some impact on eventual T1D diagnosis is the seasonality of birth. The SEARCH study showed patients that were born between the months of April through July were disproportionately diagnosed with T1D at higher rates. Furthermore, those born during November through February showed decreased rates [1]. Of note, this phenomenon was only detected in locations with more distinct seasonality (ie, higher latitudes). Exact mechanisms explaining this trend remain undetermined but hypotheses involving sunlight exposure have been proposed.

PATHOPHYSIOLOGY

The pathophysiology of T1D involves autoimmune destruction of the beta cells of the pancreas in the setting of genetic susceptibility. To date, more than 40 susceptibility genes have been identified [5]. Polymorphisms of histocompatibility loci antigens (human leukocyte antigens [HLAs]) DR and DQ, which are located on chromosome 6, contribute to up to 50% of familial cases of T1D [6]. Precipitating events that may trigger autoimmunity have been hypothesized to include viral infections, or environmental exposures to nitrosamines or cow's milk. The immune process against islet cells involves activation of T cells expressing HLA-DR, islet cell antibodies, insulin autoantibodies (IAAs), glutamic acid decarboxylase (GAD) antibodies, and islet antigen 2. Lack of self-antigen recognition is thought to mediate the autoimmune response. Clinical manifestations of T1D present when at least 90% of the beta-cell mass of the pancreas has been destroyed, and insulin deficiency occurs, presenting first as a defect in insulin secretion in response to glucose intake. Peripheral glucose uptake by the organs is reduced, and lack of insulin signaling ultimately results in a catabolic state featuring unregulated proteolysis and gluconeogenesis, lipolysis, and ketone body formation (diabetic ketoacidosis). The high osmotic load from the presence of glucose and ketones can lead to urinary losses of volume and cations ($Na+$, $K+$, P) resulting in dehydration and electrolyte depletion.

In contrast with T1D, type 2 diabetes (T2D) does not feature islet cell autoimmunity and lacks the autoantibodies found in T1D. T2D is associated with obesity, and is characterized by insulin resistance with a relative deficiency in insulin secretion. Evidence supports abnormal lipid partitioning, with lipid accumulation in muscle, liver, and visceral tissues, as contributing to insulin resistance and glucose metabolic derangements [7].

COMPLICATIONS OF DIABETES

The natural history of diabetes and the outcomes that result from poor blood glucose control are well described, including retinopathy, nephropathy, neuropathy, and cardiovascular disease. Following the discovery of insulin in 1922 and implementation in the management of T1D, patients were living longer and developing multiple medical issues later in life. Evidence emerged, strongly supporting the relationship of these complications to long-standing hyperglycemia, as shown by the Diabetes Control and Complications Trial (DCCT) and the Epidemiology of Diabetes Interventions and Complications (EDIC) follow-up. This study followed 1441 patients with T1D with an average of more than 6.5 years and assessed glycemic control and development of complications in patients managing their T1D with conventional insulin therapy versus more intensive therapy. Results showed a median glycosylated hemoglobin value of 9% in the conventional therapy group compared with 7% in the intensive therapy group. Furthermore, a substantial decrease in early-stage complications was noted in the intensive therapy group [8,9]. Analyses on youth with T1D for at least 5 years in the SEARCH study showed a 7%

prevalence (n = 1734) of diabetic neuropathy [10], 17% prevalence (n = 222) of diabetic retinopathy [11], and a 6.8% prevalence of albuminuria (n = 1316) [12]. Among 1734 subjects with T1D with normal non–high-density lipoprotein lipid measurements at baseline, 19% showed progression to dyslipidemia after follow-up of ~7 years [13].

Although multiple body systems are affected by diabetes, the organs predominantly involved include the vasculature, nerves, eyes, heart, and kidneys [14]. These complications can broadly be broken down into microvascular versus macrovascular changes. Microvascular changes include thickening of the vessel basement membrane of arterioles, capillaries, and venules, compromising vital functions such substrate delivery, oxygen exchange, and wound healing. Clinically evident changes develop over time in susceptible tissues such as the myocardium, retina, and glomeruli, which may lead to chronic hypertension. Over time, major morbidity may result from severe outcomes, including loss of eyesight, chronic kidney disease, and diabetic peripheral neuropathy, which may require subsequent limb amputation [8].

Macrovascular complications relate more to peripheral artery disease and atherosclerosis. Patients with T1D are much more likely to have an ischemic event compared with the general population. Through a variety of mechanisms, hyperglycemia causes a continuous low-grade inflammation that leads to remodeling of vessel walls and predisposition for plaque formation, enlargement, and rupture. These complications put T1D patients at risk for developing life-threatening or debilitating sequelae such as myocardial infarctions and strokes [14]. Even before the occurrence of these major events, perfusion of limbs (and especially the feet) can be compromised, resulting in ischemic pain that can be severely limiting for patients. Because of significant macrovascular disease, nearly two-thirds of patients with T1D end up dying of cardiovascular complications.

Because of these complications, early screening is vital. Fundus photography of sufficient quality is feasible among children [15]. Retinal photography has been shown to be accessible and scalable in increasing the rate of retinal screening among patients with diabetes [16]. Screening for urine microalbuminuria is recommended annually, beginning 5 years after diagnosis of T1D. If detected, treatment involves angiotensin-converting enzyme (ACE) inhibitors, although the evidence for use in adolescents is largely based on consensus from adult data [17,18]. Screening for dyslipidemia is recommended because it is often associated with poor blood glucose control. Similar to use of ACE inhibitors, there is currently insufficient evidence for statin use in children and adolescents with T1D [19], although there are studies showing potential good adherence if prescribed [20].

In addition to considering the complications discussed earlier, pregnant women with diabetes, including T1D, need to be particularly diligent about maintaining good glycemic control. Known fetal complications of maternal diabetes include miscarriage, stillbirth, premature delivery, and birth defects. Potential birth defects can involve several organ systems, such as the cardiovascular, nervous system, genitourinary, and skeletal systems. In addition, babies born to mothers with diabetes can be macrosomic and have transient hypoglycemia that may require intervention in the newborn period. Therefore, it is paramount that pregnant patients with T1D are closely followed by an endocrinologist and obstetrician concurrently to avoid complications.

MANAGEMENT

Management of T1D is a lifelong process and often requires a multidisciplinary team of medical professionals [21]. Endocrinologists, dieticians, psychologists, nursing diabetes educators, and parents are some of the key players who can contribute to adequate long-term blood glucose control in children with T1D. The goal of management should be to promote physiologic growth and maturation, and to prevent the long-term complications related to morbidity and mortality from the disease. These outcomes are highly correlated with glycemic control. Therefore, caring for patients with T1D requires maintaining balance between tightly maintaining euglycemic levels and preventing symptomatic hypoglycemic events. This balance is predominantly achieved through exogenous insulin administration, dietary modification, and physical activity.

Nearly the entirety of pharmacotherapy related to the treatment of T1D is insulin, because the pancreas cannot produce its own following destruction of the pancreatic beta cells. Insulin was discovered in the 1920s by surgeon Frederick Banting and his research assistant Charles Best, with sponsorship from physiologist J.J.R. Macleod. Before this, diabetes was a known disease entity with no treatment, resulting in hyperglycemia, glucosuria, and ketosis, which led to coma and eventually death. Attempts at dietary carbohydrate restriction delayed morbidity and mortality but did not alter the eventual outcome. In 1921, Banting ligated the pancreatic ducts of dogs, resulting in the development of diabetes. Extraction of the pancreatic islet cell secretions and reinjection into the dogs decreased blood glucose levels [22]. Collaboration with biochemist J.B. Collip led to improved purification of this insulin extract. The following year, in 1922, the insulin extract was injected into the first human patient. More patients followed, all showing decrease of blood glucose level and reversal of the ketotic process [22]. Since then, exogenous insulin has become the mainstay of T1D treatment and has allowed patients to live longer, fuller lives.

The other pillar in the approach to outpatient T1D management is maintaining a healthy diet and engaging in routine exercise [17]. Monitoring and quantification of dietary intake of carbohydrates is paramount to appropriate dosage of insulin. One skill essential for patients with T1D to master is the accurate counting of carbohydrates so that they can cover their meals with the requisite amount of insulin. Appropriate administration of exogenous insulin can mimic the physiologic response and successfully maintain euglycemia during and following meals. Consistency in carbohydrate intake simplifies the process and results in fewer dosing errors. Furthermore, maintaining an active lifestyle and participating in routine exercise decreases the body's overall need for insulin. This decreased need is accomplished through an increased sensitivity to insulin, as well as direct use of glucose by muscle tissue independent of insulin during times of peak activity. Therefore, encouraging a healthy lifestyle coupled with an appropriate insulin regimen is key to supporting patients with T1D in the promotion of optimal long-term outcomes.

TYPES OF INSULIN

Since the initial discovery, research into insulin has led to development of different types of insulin with unique pharmacokinetic and pharmacodynamic profiles. Insulin therapy is delivered by subcutaneous injection because gastrointestinal enzymes digest peptides taken orally. Led by Banting's example, insulin that was used to treat T1D was historically of animal origin, typically bovine or porcine. However, in the 1980s, recombinant DNA technology allowed human insulin to be synthesized in vitro, which led to a decline in the use of animal insulin. Modification of the recombinant peptides to form analogues confers changes to pharmacodynamic properties, resulting in various formulations that attempt to closely mimic natural physiology. Insulin is broadly grouped into categories based on the onset, peak, and duration of action, and is typically classified as either rapid, short, intermediate, or long acting [23]. These types of insulin are used in combination for the 3 components of insulin delivery: to cover carbohydrate intake, to correct high blood glucose levels, and to provide basal insulin to keep blood glucose level stable during periods of fasting. Table 1 summarizes the types of insulin and the available forms.

Rapid-acting insulin

Rapid-acting insulin formulations available in the United States include lispro, aspart, and glulisine, created through amino acid substitutions in the insulin peptide chains. These formulations achieve their desired effect when administered subcutaneously, because intravenous injection leads to a delay in onset of action and results in an effect more closely resembling regular (short-acting) insulin. Onset of rapid-acting insulin is within 15 minutes and peak effect occurs around 1 hour. Duration can be between 3 to 5 hours. Because of its quick onset and peak time, rapid-acting insulin is typically used prandially as a bolus to cover any ingested carbohydrates. It can also be used as correction to help decrease blood glucose levels if hyperglycemia occurs. Rapid-acting insulin is available in vials, cartridges for a reusable pen device, or in disposable pens, and is the only class of insulin currently approved for use in personal insulin pumps [23,24].

Rapid-acting insulin as a powder for inhalation was approved for use in 2006 as an alternative to injection [25]. However, because of concerns about impact on pulmonary function, this human insulin (recombinant DNA origin; marketed as Exubera) was minimally used by patients and providers and, thus,

Table 1
Types of insulin and their profiles of action

Type	Onset of action	Peak effect	Duration of action
Rapid-acting analogues			
Lispro, aspart, glulisine	Within 15 min	1–2 h	4–6 h
Faster-acting aspart	Within 15 min	1–2 h	4–6 h
Powder for inhalation	Within 15 min	30 min	3 h
Short-acting analogues			
Regular	Within 30–60 min	2–4 h	6–8 h
Intermediate-acting analogues (zinc or protamine)			
NPH	1.5–2.5 h	4–6 h	12–18 h
Long-acting analogues			
Glargine	70 min	None	22–24 h
Detemir	1.5–2.5 h	None	12–24 h
Degludec	1–4 h	None	Up to 42 h
Premixed	Premixed ratios		
NPH/regular	70% NPH, 30% regular insulin		
Protamine-aspart/aspart	70% protamine-aspart and 30% insulin aspart		
Protamine-lispro/lispro	70% protamine-lispro and 30% insulin lispro		
	75% protamine-lispro and 25% insulin lispro		
	50% protamine-lispro and 50% insulin lispro		

Abbreviation: NPH, neutral protamine Hagedorn.

was taken off the market the year following its introduction. In 2014, another rapid-acting powder for inhalation was US Food and Drug Administration (FDA) approved and remains available today (Afrezza). It is currently approved for use in adults with T1D in combination with long-acting insulin, or in adults with T2D. Its challenges include inflexible dosing, and contraindication in chronic lung disease because of risk of bronchospasm.

Short-acting insulin

Short-acting insulin is the term given to regular human insulin. Its onset occurs within 1 hour and it peaks around 2 to 4 hours, with a duration of action as long as 8 hours. With the delay in onset of action, preprandial regular insulin injected subcutaneously is therefore recommended to be given about 30 minutes before a meal to align with food absorption. However, when delivered intravenously, regular insulin is rapid acting, and therefore is the insulin of choice for insulin infusion (insulin drip) during management of diabetic ketoacidosis.

Intermediate-acting insulin

Intermediate-acting isophane insulin is also known as NPH (neutral protamine Hagedorn) because it consists of regular insulin combined with protamine that serves to slow subcutaneous absorption. NPH was created early along the insulin timeline, back in 1936. The onset of action is 1 to 2 hours, with peak activity around 4 to 10 hours and a total duration of more than 14 hours. In T1D, NPH is primarily administered in combination with a rapid-acting or short-acting prandial insulin. Formulations of 70%/30% premixed insulin are commercially available as NPH/regular, or protamine/rapid-acting combinations, along with 50%/50% protamine/rapid-acting and 75%/25% protamine/rapid-acting mixtures. Although the fixed ratios may be less physiologic and do not facilitate adjustment to correct acutely for high blood sugar levels, these regimens may be considered for patients who have trouble with adherence. NPH, as well as these mixtures, are available in vials, cartridges, and disposable pens [23].

Long-acting insulin

Long-acting insulins are analogues designed to have a delayed pharmacodynamic profile and thus are used as basal insulins. Their sustained action serves to downregulate gluconeogenesis in the liver and prevent ketosis in patients with T1D. Three types of long-acting insulin for subcutaneous injection exist on the market in the United States: detemir, glargine, and degludec. Detemir has a myristic acid attached to lysine at the B chain position 29 (B29), with a deletion of B30, and has an onset of action within 3 to 4 hours [26]. Glargine has 2 arginine residues added at the end of the B chain at B31 and B32, and a substitution of glycine for asparagine at position A21, with an onset of action as early as 90 minutes. Both detemir and glargine have a duration of action up to 24 hours. Degludec, a newer analogue (deletion of B30, with a palmitic acid attached to a γ-L-glutamic acid on B29), has onset after about 1 hour but can last up to 42 hours, the long duration of which confers possible benefits as a basal insulin [27–29]. In general, all long-acting preparations have a steady effect and minimal peak. Given these properties, long-acting insulins are typically given once daily in combination with prandial rapid-acting or short-acting insulin. In the treatment of T1D, the exception to needing long-acting insulin is when using an insulin pump. Because pumps constantly infuse rapid-acting insulin (basal rate), these patients do not require use of a long-acting formulation.

INSULIN PUMPS

Insulin pumps deliver continuous subcutaneous insulin infusion, and were first used in the 1970s as an alternative to multiple daily injections [30,31]. Initial models were simple, only allowing a fixed basal infusion rate and requiring manual input of total units of insulin for additional boluses during mealtime or correction. Since its commercialization, there have been many advances in the functionality and capability of these devices, especially in recent years [32,33]. Insulin pumps are now more sophisticated and allow for customization, as well as some autonomous adjustments depending on current or predicted blood glucose levels. Furthermore, studies have compared patients on pumps with those on intensive injections and have established clear benefit. A 2002 meta-analysis of 13 randomized controlled trials concluded that patients on insulin pumps have a significantly lower average blood glucose level, lower glycosylated hemoglobin value, and required less overall total daily insulin than those using traditional injections [34]. Among children with T1D, use of insulin pumps resulted in significantly better long-term blood glucose control up to 6 years compared with multiple daily injections [35].

The basic functionality of the insulin pump is to provide a continuous subcutaneous infusion of rapid-acting insulin and negate the need for separate basal insulin (Table 2 provides a glossary of terms used in insulin pump technology). Pumps can now be programmed to have multiple basal rates, depending on activity level. For example, insulin requirements during exercise decrease because there is enhanced uptake of glucose directly into muscles and therefore decreasing the basal rate of insulin may prevent a hypoglycemic episode. In contrast, during sleep, there is comparatively low glucose use, but increasing the basal rate can help attenuate hyperglycemia from the dawn phenomenon. In addition to basal delivery, bolus insulin is given to cover meals and for correction of increased blood glucose levels. Patient-specific insulin to carbohydrate ratios can be preset and doses are automatically calculated by input of the total amount of planned carbohydrates into the pump. In addition, patient-specific correction factors (insulin sensitivity factor) and blood glucose targets are programmed so that hyperglycemia can be corrected appropriately. The pump also tracks active insulin on board in order to prevent hypoglycemia from insulin stacking if doses are given too close together in time. Some pumps also have options for alternate settings for exercise and sleep when insulin delivery needs change. Because all insulin is administered through a single device, patients experience fewer invasive events compared with multiple daily injections. In addition, extra snacks, seconds on a meal, or dessert can be covered by insulin via the pump without an additional injection, thereby facilitating adherence. A typical insulin pump infusion set or patch can be used up to 3 days before it needs to be changed, ideally rotated to minimize known injection site side effects such as lipohypertrophy.

Another major way in which modern pumps differ from their predecessors is their outward appearance and size. Across the decades, pumps have become smaller. They were initially large and bulky, but now approximate the size of a deck of playing cards [32]. Pumps in the United States are now divided into traditional pumps, and patch pumps. A traditional insulin pump is tethered to the injection site by a length of tubing. The pump can be stored within clothing or a pouch and has buttons and a screen that are used to control insulin delivery. These pumps are typically not waterproof and must be disconnected before bathing or water submersion. In contrast, patch insulin pumps adhere the insulin reservoir directly to the patient's skin. These pumps are waterproof and are usually controlled remotely by a separate device [33].

Despite all the evidence showing the benefits of pump use, there are still disadvantages to consider. A patient using a pump is attached to the delivery system constantly. Insulin pump hardware may malfunction for a variety of reasons. Tubing obstruction from flattening and bending can occur, or unintentional disconnection of a pump site. Either of these situations can lead to a lapse in insulin delivery, which can rapidly progress to hyperglycemia and potentially ketoacidosis. Therefore, it is always recommended that a manual option

Table 2
Insulin delivery system technology: glossary of terms

Term	Definition
Closed-loop system or artificial pancreas	A coordinated system of devices that includes a glucose sensor, a control algorithm, and an insulin pump that continuously automates insulin delivery based on the blood glucose levels
Hybrid closed-loop system	A coordinated system of devices that includes a glucose sensor, a control algorithm, and an insulin pump that partially automates insulin delivery. Current models automate basal delivery, with emergence of ability to automate correctional insulin dosing. Still requires manual entry of carbohydrate intake
Control algorithm	A key element of the above systems involving computational models to monitor glucose fluctuations and calculate the rate of insulin to be delivered every few minutes
CGM	A system that constantly monitors a person's glucose values via a glucose sensor and wirelessly transmits a reading every few minutes to a display device. Real-time CGM constantly transmits data, while intermittently scanned CGM requires waving a receiver over the sensor in order to obtain the data
Sensor	The part of the CGM that is inserted subcutaneously to measure interstitial glucose concentrations. Electrodes in the sensor measure the electrical current generated by enzymatic reactions of glucose
Transmitter	The part of the CGM that is attached to the sensor and wirelessly sends the glucose measurement to a receiving device for display
Receiver/display device	A handheld device that receives the glucose values and displays them for review. In some models, this is integrated into the patient's own mobile phone device
Insulin pump	A computerized, battery-operated device that delivers rapid-acting insulin subcutaneously through a catheter. The pump is programmed to deliver insulin continuously at desired basal rates and is directed to deliver bolus insulin for mealtime coverage and/or correction. Traditional pumps store the insulin in a reservoir and deliver it through an infusion set that includes a length of tubing. Patch pumps are smaller than traditional pumps and attach to the skin for direct insulin delivery from the reservoir through a subcutaneous cannula, without lengthy tubing. A separate handheld device is used to program the basal rates and boluses

(*continued on next page*)

Table 2
(*continued*)

Term	Definition
Infusion set	The insulin pump parts that deliver insulin from the device to the subcutaneous tissue. Includes a small cannula inserted under the skin manually or through use of an autoinjection device. Involves connection to the pump by a length of catheter tubing. Generally needs to be changed every 3 d
Reservoir	The component of the insulin pump that stores the insulin in the device for infusion. In traditional pumps, the reservoir is filled and loaded into the pump. In patch pumps, the reservoir is part of the patch and has a port to load insulin before use

Abbreviation: CGM, continuous glucose monitor.

of injecting insulin be available, such as a pen or vial and syringe. Furthermore, an insulin pump can ease the management of diabetes but does not eliminate the need for patient-guided control, and so expectations for benefits and disadvantages should be discussed with patients before initiation [33].

In the last 5 years, pump technology has continued to advance, allowing increasingly automated modification of insulin delivery. Many commercially available pumps can now interface with a continuous glucose monitor (CGM) to interpret and react to a patient's serum glucose levels in real time using a control algorithm. These advanced systems are discussed later.

CONTINUOUS GLUCOSE MONITORING

The newest insulin pump designs with autonomous basal rate regulation would not be possible without the existence of continuous glucose monitoring. Current CGM technology uses the glucose-oxidation reaction to convert measured interstitial glucose levels into an electrical signal and transmits the signal to a receiving device [36]. It does this from a small filament that is inserted into the subcutaneous tissue, commonly on the abdomen, deltoid, or gluteal region. From this, glucose values are generated in real time and can provide the patient or clinician with a substantial amount of data about serum blood sugar trends that can help to guide management. Advantages include decreasing the frequency of finger-stick blood sampling for comprehensive management of T1D.

CGM was first FDA approved for use by health care professionals in the United States in 1999, but early methods of measuring serum glucose were constrained by how accurate their readings were. In 2004, the first CGM was approved for personal use (Medtronic Real-Time Guardian) [36], followed by models from companies such as Dexcom Inc and Abbott Diabetes Care, but they still had accuracy challenges, requiring frequent calibration with finger-stick blood glucose monitoring as well. In the last decade, in each new generation of CGM devices, accuracy has improved to approximate traditional methods of glucose measurement. Recent models have moved toward no requirement for calibration [37], including the Dexcom G5 and G6, and the Abbott Freestyle Libre. (The Freestyle Libre is considered an intermittently scanned CGM, requiring the wearer to move a receiver over the sensor in order to obtain data, and can be worn for up to 2 weeks at a time before needing to be changed.) CGM has even been configured to communicate with smartphones so as to eliminate the need to carry around a separate transmitting device. The comfort and size of the newer sensors have also continued to improve, making them a much more appealing option than first-generation CGMs [36]. The FDA has recently approved an implantable CGM device. About the size of a pea, it is inserted into the upper arm, where it can remain for up to 90 days. Accuracy is comparable with other current CGMs but does require a procedure to implant and continued daily calibration [38]. Suffice it to say, CGM technology has advanced significantly since its introduction 2 decades ago.

Although the data regarding CGM use were initially mixed, as time has elapsed there has been a demonstrable benefit identified in those patients using it. The Juvenile Diabetes Research Foundation Continuous Glucose Monitoring Study Group released several prominent studies from 2008 to 2010 that greatly advocated for the use of CGM [39–41]. Findings overall supported a substantial decrease in glycosylated hemoglobin value in patients using CGM across all ages, and also minimized the frequency of hypoglycemic episodes by 33% to 50% [42]. Subsequent studies have duplicated and confirmed these results, leading to the widespread adoption of CGM into T1D management practice.

Even with all the advances of CGM since its inception, there still remain some notable limitations. The glucose-oxidation reaction that CGM relies on can be interfered with by several common medications, such as acetaminophen and ascorbate. In addition, subcutaneous glucose measurement may differ in real time from serum and so values noted on the transmitter are not perfectly reflective of actual blood glucose value. Although only 5 to 10 minutes, this delay has the potential to affect real-time decisions during hypoglycemia or hyperglycemia episodes [36]. One emerging area for improvement is cybersecurity [43]. If hacked, malicious excess insulin delivery leading to hypoglycemia or underinsulinization leading to diabetic ketoacidosis may occur. Personal blood glucose data are a Health Insurance Portability and Accountability Act (HIPAA)–protected quantity, so more advanced measures to protect this information require further research.

CLOSED-LOOP SYSTEMS/ARTIFICIAL PANCREAS

A closed-loop system is the current goal in insulin delivery technology, which is essentially creating an artificial pancreas. A closed-loop system refers to a fully automated system in which a glucose sensor transmits the glucose value and its trajectory to a control algorithm, which then calculates the amount of insulin required and instructs the insulin pump to deliver insulin accordingly. These systems aim to minimize low blood glucose level occurrences and increase the time the patient spends in the target blood glucose range. At the present time, the systems available for clinical care are hybrid closed-loop systems, because they can automate basal insulin delivery, but still require manual entry of carbohydrate intake and manual direction to deliver correctional doses of insulin. From the technology development standpoint, 1 significant challenge in advancement of these systems is addressing the time delay between glucose sensing and adjustment of rate/amount of insulin delivery. The patients may also experience challenges with implementation, such as problems with the sensor or inconsistent ability to stay in the automatic mode [44]. Recent clinical trials show promising models in development [45–47]. One new model tested among adolescents with T1D [48,49] is able to automate correctional insulin delivery in addition to the basal and has recently gained FDA approval for use.

PREVENTION OF TYPE 1 DIABETES

Prevention of T1D has been explored for decades, but has not yet yielded a successful intervention. Prevention can be broken down into primary, secondary, and tertiary prevention. Many studies have been conducted through the international T1D TrialNet study network. Primary prevention is the attempt to deter or delay development of T1D in susceptible patients. Studies have examined how environmental changes such as dietary exposure might modulate development of T1D [50] in at-risk patients with a strong family history or high-risk HLA genotype. Various elimination diets, such as avoidance of cow's milk or gluten, among high-risk infants ultimately did not prevent T1D compared with patients on unrestricted diets [51,52]. Other trials examined nutritional supplementation and the impact on autoimmunity in those at risk. Vitamin D, omega 3 fatty acids [53], and so-called viral vaccines (given the relationship between certain enterovirus infections) are just some examples of interventions that have been studied [54] without any evidence of effectiveness. At the present time, there are no effective means of primary prevention.

Secondary prevention is halting the progression from detection of markers of autoimmunity to development of clinical disease. Individuals with increasing numbers of islet antibodies are at progressively higher risk of developing T1D. Those with 2 or more antibodies had a 70% risk of being diagnosed with T1D within 10 years, whereas this percentage is 14.5% in those with a single autoantibody and less than 1% for those with none [55]. Because these autoantibodies can be identified years before clinical criteria for a diagnosis of T1D are met, researchers have attempted to intervene in this window and either slow or prevent the progression to complete exogenous insulin dependence. Parenteral, oral, and even intranasal insulin have been studied in clinical trials to observe for preservation of beta-cell function [56–58]. Most of the results have been disappointing, but some evidence suggests that oral insulin can delay a diagnosis by nearly 5 years in patients with multiple autoantibodies, especially in those with high IAA titers [56]. Other agents, including nicotinamide [59], abatacept (cytotoxic T lymphocyte–associated protein 4

[CTLA-4] immunoglobulin) [60], GAD, and several monoclonal antibodies, have also been studied in clinical trials with some suggestion that treatment can slow the decline in beta-cell function, but they do not prevent progression of disease.

Preserving beta-cell function and thereby endogenous insulin production as long as possible in individuals with newly diagnosed diabetes is the goal of tertiary prevention. Typically, management requires less insulin initially after diagnosis because of residual beta-cell activity, which is known as the honeymoon phase. Prolongation of this period would serve to decrease exogenous insulin requirement and promote better-controlled blood glucose levels. C-peptide has been used as a marker for continued beta-cell function throughout the honeymoon phase. Study subjects have been reported to experience lower rates of long-term complications when they have sustained measurable C-peptide levels [61]. Past studies examined the potential for remission after treatment with immunosuppressants such as cyclosporine, prednisone, and azathioprine [62–64]. In recent years, more targeted therapies have been studied in order to avoid the systemic side effects experienced with those agents. Many antigens and monoclonal antibodies (eg, teplizumab, otelixizumab, rituximab) have been studied for tertiary prevention, some with moderate evidence in maintaining C-peptide detection [65,66]. Trials on treatments targeting innate immunity are also in progress [67]. However, there is currently insufficient evidence to promote any particular treatment, but further studies in prevention remain a priority in T1D research.

ISLET CELL TRANSPLANT

Transplant of islet cells is a major area of research for a potential cure for T1D. The aim of transplanting physiologically active islet cells is to achieve insulin independence. However, implementation has proved difficult, with major challenges being the autoimmune nature of the disease and limitation of available islet cells. At present, islet cell transplant is available as an experimental therapy in adults with T1D who have hypoglycemic unawareness and/or glycemic lability despite adequate insulin treatment.

Islet cell transplant involves infusion of islet cells isolated from 1 or more deceased donors into the portal vein of the transplant recipient. More than 1 infusion may be necessary to deliver enough islet cells for the recipient to become insulin independent. The recipient must take immunosuppressant medication to prevent transplant rejection. Initial studies to implant islet cells yielded inconsistent results and only transiently achieved insulin independence. From 1990 to 1999, of a total of 267 transplant recipients, only 8.2% sustained insulin independence 1 year posttransplant [68]. Establishment of the Edmonton protocol using the immunosuppressive regimen including sirolimus, tacrolimus, and the anti-CD25 antibody daclizumab resulted in 7 patients living independent of exogenous insulin after 1 year posttransplant [69]. This success was followed by additional transplants performed internationally reporting positive results, with 16 patients (44%)

showing insulin independence for 1 year, and 5 (10%) of these patients showing this benefit up to 2 years [70]. Notable limitations to transplant include the burden of islet cells required to attain insulin independence, which requires multiple donors. Further work has included identification of factors related to single-donor transplant success, such as low preoperative insulin requirements [71]. Although not all transplant recipients meet the primary end points of insulin independence at 1 year, C-peptide levels may still be higher than pretransplant, which allows improved blood glucose control and the potential for lower insulin doses.

Because of the shortage of islet cell donors, alternative cell types have been investigated as possibilities for implantation. Pluripotent stem cells and pancreatic nonendocrine cells have recently been identified as front-running candidates for this purpose [72]. However, even as research progresses toward finding a sustainable method of creating functional replicants of islet cells, the barrier of autoimmunity still looms. Other research has explored ways to protect and preserve implanted cells so that they do not have the same fate as the native beta cells. Studies include using human pancreatic progenitor cells created in vitro that mature into functional beta cells after implantation. If efficacious, synthetically derived cells would eliminate the burden of relying on donor islet cells and thereby greatly increase their availability. Moreover, development of an encapsulation device may serve to protect the implanted cells from host immune cells, which could circumvent the need for long-term immunosuppression [73,74]. Although these trials and products still remain in the early stages, further advances are poised to revolutionize T1D treatment.

SUMMARY

T1D is a disease that affects millions of people throughout the world. Significant morbidity and mortality result in those with long-standing, poorly controlled T1D. Therefore, empowering children and adolescents with T1D to maintain tight glycemic control early is paramount to helping them avoid microvascular and macrovascular complications later in life. For this reason, the development of new technology to aid in the achievement of this goal has been critical. Over the decades, new forms of recombinant insulin have allowed more physiologic regimens to help approximate the function of native beta cells. Insulin pumps with a basal rate have helped to more accurately mimic healthy pancreatic function, as well as reduce frequency of daily injections for patients. CGM technology has provided substantial data for patients and providers to guide insulin therapy, and has allowed closed-loop systems that act as an artificial pancreas by autonomously modifying insulin delivery based on blood glucose trends. Research into prevention and potential curative measures such as islet cell transplant are ongoing and could lead to disease-modifying advances in T1D management. Although advances have been gradual in the search for a cure, the future remains bright for T1D research, which has the potential to improve the lives of millions of patients worldwide.

Disclosure

The authors have nothing to disclose.

References

[1] International Diabetes Federation. IDF Diabetes Atlas. 9th edn. Brussels, Belgium: International Diabetes Federation; 2019.
[2] Hamman RF, Bell RA, Dabelea D, et al. The SEARCH for diabetes in youth study: rationale, findings, and future directions. Diabetes Care 2014;37(12):3336–44.
[3] Karvonen M, Viik-Kajander M, Moltchanova E, et al. Incidence of childhood type 1 diabetes worldwide. Diabetes Mondiale (DiaMond) Project Group. Diabetes Care 2000;23(10): 1516–26.
[4] Maahs DM, West NA, Lawrence JM, et al. Epidemiology of type 1 diabetes. Endocrinol Metab Clin North Am 2010;39(3):481–97.
[5] Barrett JC, Clayton DG, Concannon P, et al. Genome-wide association study and meta-analysis find that over 40 loci affect risk of type 1 diabetes. Nat Genet 2009;41(6):703–7.
[6] Noble JA, Valdes AM. Genetics of the HLA region in the prediction of type 1 diabetes. Curr Diabetes Rep 2011;11(6):533–42.
[7] D'Adamo E, Caprio S. Type 2 diabetes in youth: epidemiology and pathophysiology. Diabetes Care 2011;34(Suppl 2):S161–5.
[8] Nathan DM. The diabetes control and complications trial/epidemiology of diabetes interventions and complications study at 30 years: overview. Diabetes Care 2014;37(1):9–16.
[9] The relationship of glycemic exposure (HbA1c) to the risk of development and progression of retinopathy in the diabetes control and complications trial. Diabetes 1995;44(8): 968–83.
[10] Jaiswal M, Divers J, Dabelea D, et al. Prevalence of and risk factors for diabetic peripheral neuropathy in youth with type 1 and type 2 diabetes: search for diabetes in youth study. Diabetes Care 2017;40(9):1226–332.
[11] Mayer-Davis EJ, Davis C, Saadine J, et al. Diabetic retinopathy in the SEARCH for Diabetes in Youth Cohort: a pilot study. Diabet Med 2012;29(9):1148–52.
[12] Kahkoska AR, Isom S, Divers J, et al. The early natural history of albuminuria in young adults with youth-onset type 1 and type 2 diabetes. J Diabetes Complications 2018;32(12): 1160–8.
[13] Shah AS, Maahs DM, Stafford JM, et al. Predictors of dyslipidemia over time in youth with type 1 diabetes: for the SEARCH for diabetes in youth study. Diabetes Care 2017;40(4): 607–13.
[14] Chawla A, Chawla R, Jaggi S. Microvasular and macrovascular complications in diabetes mellitus: distinct or continuum? Indian J Endocrinol Metab 2016;20(4):546–51.
[15] Toffoli D, Bruce BB, Lamirel C, et al. Feasibility and quality of nonmydriatic fundus photography in children. J AAPOS 2011;15(6):567–72.
[16] Daskivich LP, Vasquez C, Martinez C Jr, et al. Implementation and evaluation of a large-scale teleretinal diabetic retinopathy screening program in the Los Angeles county department of health services. JAMA Intern Med 2017;177(5):642–9.
[17] Chiang JL, Maahs DM, Garvey KC, et al. Type 1 diabetes in children and adolescents: a position statement by the American Diabetes Association. Diabetes Care 2018;41(9): 2026–44.
[18] Marcovecchio ML, Chiesa ST, Bond S, et al. ACE inhibitors and statins in adolescents with type 1 diabetes. N Engl J Med 2017;377(18):1733–45.
[19] Gourgari E, Stafford JM, D'Agostino R Jr, et al. Association of metformin and statin medications with surrogate measures of cardiovascular disease in youth with type 1 diabetes: the SEARCH for diabetes in youth study. Ann Pediatr Endocrinol Metab 2019;24(3):187–94.
[20] Niechcial E, Acerini CL, Chiesa ST, et al. Medication adherence during adjunct therapy with statins and ACE inhibitors in adolescents with type 1 diabetes. Diabetes Care 2020;43(5): 1070–6.

[21] Children and adolescents: standards of medical care in diabetes-2020. Diabetes Care 2020;43(Suppl 1):S163–82.
[22] Banting FG, Best CH, Collip JB, et al. Pancreatic extracts in the treatment of diabetes mellitus. Can Med Assoc J 1922;12(3):141–6.
[23] Donner T, Sarkar S. Insulin - pharmacology, therapeutic regimens, and principles of intensive insulin therapy. In: Feingold KR, Anawalt B, Boyce A, et al, editors. Endotext. South Dartmouth (MA): MDText.com, Inc; 2019.
[24] Weinzimer SA, Ternand C, Howard C, et al. A randomized trial comparing continuous subcutaneous insulin infusion of insulin aspart versus insulin lispro in children and adolescents with type 1 diabetes. Diabetes Care 2008;31(2):210–5.
[25] Oleck J, Kassam S, Goldman JD. Commentary: why was inhaled insulin a failure in the market? Diabetes Spectr 2016;29(3):180–4.
[26] Tibaldi JM. Evolution of insulin: from human to analog. Am J Med 2014;127(10 Suppl): S25–38.
[27] Schmitt J, Scott ML. Insulin Degludec in adolescents with type 1 diabetes: is newer better? - A retrospective self-control case series in adolescents with a history of diabetic ketoacidosis. Horm Res Paediatr 2019;92(3):179–85.
[28] Elahi S, Patel AD, Guandalini C, et al. Impact of switching youth with diabetes to insulin degludec in clinical practice. Endocr Pract 2019;25(3):226–9.
[29] Lane W, Bailey TS, Gerety G, et al. Effect of insulin Degludec vs insulin glargine U100 on hypoglycemia in patients with type 1 diabetes: the SWITCH 1 randomized clinical trial. JAMA 2017;318(1):33–44.
[30] Tamborlane WV, Sherwin RS, Genel M, et al. Reduction to normal of plasma glucose in juvenile diabetes by subcutaneous administration of insulin with a portable infusion pump. N Engl J Med 1979;300(11):573–8.
[31] Pickup JC, Keen H, Parsons JA, et al. Continuous subcutaneous insulin infusion: an approach to achieving normoglycaemia. Br Med J 1978;1(6107):204–7.
[32] Paldus B, Lee MH, O'Neal DN. Insulin pumps in general practice. Aust prescriber 2018;41(6):186–90.
[33] Sora ND, Shashpal F, Bond EA, et al. Insulin pumps: review of technological advancement in diabetes management. Am J Med Sci 2019;358(5):326–31.
[34] Pickup J, Mattock M, Kerry S. Glycaemic control with continuous subcutaneous insulin infusion compared with intensive insulin injections in patients with type 1 diabetes: meta-analysis of randomised controlled trials. BMJ 2002;324(7339):705.
[35] Burckhardt MA, Smith GJ, Cooper MN, et al. Real-world outcomes of insulin pump compared to injection therapy in a population-based sample of children with type 1 diabetes. Pediatr Diabetes 2018;19(8):1459–66.
[36] Cappon G, Vettoretti M, Sparacino G, et al. Continuous glucose monitoring sensors for diabetes management: a review of technologies and applications. Diabetes Metab J 2019;43(4):383–97.
[37] Bailey TS. Clinical implications of accuracy measurements of continuous glucose sensors. Diabetes Technol Ther 2017;19(S2):S51–4.
[38] Deiss D, Szadkowska A, Gordon D, et al. Clinical practice recommendations on the routine use of eversense, the first long-term implantable continuous glucose monitoring system. Diabetes Technol Ther 2019;21(5):254–64.
[39] Tamborlane WV, Beck RW, Bode BW, et al. Continuous glucose monitoring and intensive treatment of type 1 diabetes. N Engl J Med 2008;359(14):1464–76.
[40] Effectiveness of continuous glucose monitoring in a clinical care environment: evidence from the Juvenile Diabetes Research Foundation continuous glucose monitoring (JDRF-CGM) trial. Diabetes Care 2010;33(1):17–22.
[41] Beck RW, Buckingham B, Miller K, et al. Factors predictive of use and of benefit from continuous glucose monitoring in type 1 diabetes. Diabetes Care 2009;32(11):1947–53.

[42] Rodbard D. Continuous glucose monitoring: a review of recent studies demonstrating improved glycemic outcomes. Diabetes Technol Ther 2017;19(S3):S25–37.
[43] Klonoff DC. Cybersecurity for connected diabetes devices. J Diabetes Sci Technol 2015;9(5):1143–7.
[44] Goodwin G, Waldman G, Lyons J, et al. OR14-5 challenges in implementing hybrid closed loop insulin pump therapy (medtronic 670g) in a 'real world' clinical setting. J Endocr Soc 2019;3(Supplement_1).
[45] Anderson SM, Dassau E, Raghinaru D, et al. The international diabetes closed-loop study: testing artificial pancreas component interoperability. Diabetes Technol Ther 2019;21(2): 73–80.
[46] Renard E, Farret A, Kropff J, et al. Day-and-night closed-loop glucose control in patients with type 1 diabetes under free-living conditions: results of a single-arm 1-month experience compared with a previously reported feasibility study of evening and night at home. Diabetes Care 2016;39(7):1151–60.
[47] Brown SA, Breton MD, Anderson SM, et al. Overnight closed-loop control improves glycemic control in a multicenter study of adults with type 1 diabetes. J Clin Endocrinol Metab 2017;102(10):3674–82.
[48] Schoelwer MJ, Robic JL, Gautier T, et al. Safety and efficacy of initializing the control-IQ artificial pancreas system based on total daily insulin in adolescents with type 1 diabetes. Diabetes Technol Ther 2020. [Epub ahead of print].
[49] Ekhlaspour L, Forlenza GP, Chernavvsky D, et al. Closed loop control in adolescents and children during winter sports: Use of the Tandem Control-IQ AP system. Pediatr Diabetes 2019;20(6):759–68.
[50] Norris JM, Barriga K, Klingensmith G, et al. Timing of initial cereal exposure in infancy and risk of islet autoimmunity. Jama 2003;290(13):1713–20.
[51] Hummel S, Pfluger M, Hummel M, et al. Primary dietary intervention study to reduce the risk of islet autoimmunity in children at increased risk for type 1 diabetes: the BABYDIET study. Diabetes Care 2011;34(6):1301–5.
[52] Knip M, Virtanen SM, Seppa K, et al. Dietary intervention in infancy and later signs of beta-cell autoimmunity. N Engl J Med 2010;363(20):1900–8.
[53] Norris JM, Yin X, Lamb MM, et al. Omega-3 polyunsaturated fatty acid intake and islet autoimmunity in children at increased risk for type 1 diabetes. Jama 2007;298(12):1420–8.
[54] Chiarelli F, Giannini C, Primavera M. Prediction and prevention of type 1 diabetes in children. Clin Pediatr Endocrinol 2019;28(3):43–57.
[55] Wherrett DK. Trials in the prevention of type 1 diabetes: current and future. Can J Diabetes 2014;38(4):279–84.
[56] Skyler JS, Krischer JP, Wolfsdorf J, et al. Effects of oral insulin in relatives of patients with type 1 diabetes: The Diabetes Prevention Trial–Type 1. Diabetes Care 2005;28(5):1068–76.
[57] Effects of insulin in relatives of patients with type 1 diabetes mellitus. N Engl J Med 2002;346(22):1685–91.
[58] Nanto-Salonen K, Kupila A, Simell S, et al. Nasal insulin to prevent type 1 diabetes in children with HLA genotypes and autoantibodies conferring increased risk of disease: a double-blind, randomised controlled trial. Lancet 2008;372(9651):1746–55.
[59] Gale EA, Bingley PJ, Emmett CL, et al. European Nicotinamide Diabetes Intervention Trial (ENDIT): a randomised controlled trial of intervention before the onset of type 1 diabetes. Lancet 2004;363(9413):925–31.
[60] Orban T, Bundy B, Becker DJ, et al. Co-stimulation modulation with abatacept in patients with recent-onset type 1 diabetes: a randomised, double-blind, placebo-controlled trial. Lancet 2011;378(9789):412–9.
[61] Steffes MW, Sibley S, Jackson M, et al. Beta-cell function and the development of diabetes-related complications in the diabetes control and complications trial. Diabetes Care 2003;26(3):832–6.

[62] Silverstein J, Maclaren N, Riley W, et al. Immunosuppression with azathioprine and prednisone in recent-onset insulin-dependent diabetes mellitus. N Engl J Med 1988;319(10): 599–604.
[63] Feutren G, Papoz L, Assan R, et al. Cyclosporin increases the rate and length of remissions in insulin-dependent diabetes of recent onset. Results of a multicentre double-blind trial. Lancet 1986;2(8499):119–24.
[64] Bougneres PF, Carel JC, Castano L, et al. Factors associated with early remission of type I diabetes in children treated with cyclosporine. N Engl J Med 1988;318(11):663–70.
[65] Aronson R, Gottlieb PA, Christiansen JS, et al. Low-dose otelixizumab anti-CD3 monoclonal antibody DEFEND-1 study: results of the randomized phase III study in recent-onset human type 1 diabetes. Diabetes Care 2014;37(10):2746–54.
[66] Demeester S, Keymeulen B, Kaufman L, et al. Preexisting insulin autoantibodies predict efficacy of otelixizumab in preserving residual beta-cell function in recent-onset type 1 diabetes. Diabetes Care 2015;38(4):644–51.
[67] Moran A, Bundy B, Becker DJ, et al. Interleukin-1 antagonism in type 1 diabetes of recent onset: two multicentre, randomised, double-blind, placebo-controlled trials. Lancet 2013;381(9881):1905–15.
[68] Shapiro AM, Lakey JR, Ryan EA, et al. Islet transplantation in seven patients with type 1 diabetes mellitus using a glucocorticoid-free immunosuppressive regimen. N Engl J Med 2000;343(4):230–8.
[69] Gamble A, Pepper AR, Bruni A, et al. The journey of islet cell transplantation and future development. Islets 2018;10(2):80–94.
[70] Shapiro AM, Ricordi C, Hering BJ, et al. International trial of the Edmonton protocol for islet transplantation. N Engl J Med 2006;355(13):1318–30.
[71] Al-Adra DP, Gill RS, Imes S, et al. Single-donor islet transplantation and long-term insulin independence in select patients with type 1 diabetes mellitus. Transplantation 2014;98(9): 1007–12.
[72] Dominguez-Bendala J, Lanzoni G, Klein D, et al. The human endocrine pancreas: new insights on replacement and regeneration. Trends Endocrinol Metab 2016;27(3):153–62.
[73] Cooper-Jones B, Ford C. Islet cell replacement therapy for insulin-dependent diabetes. CADTH issues in emerging health technologies. Ottawa (ON): Canadian Agency for Drugs and Technologies in Health Copyright (c) CADTH 2017; 2016. p. 1–9, You are permitted to reproduce this document for non-commercial purposes, provided it is not modified when reproduced and appropriate credit is given to CADTH.
[74] Agulnick AD, Ambruzs DM, Moorman MA, et al. Insulin-producing endocrine cells differentiated in vitro from human embryonic stem cells function in macroencapsulation devices in vivo. Stem Cell Transl Med 2015;4(10):1214–22.

Advances in Pediatrics 67 (2020) 93–104

ADVANCES IN PEDIATRICS

Update on Precocious Puberty

Who Should Be Treated?

Paul B. Kaplowitz, MD, PhD

Division of Endocrinology, Children's National Hospital, George Washington University School of Medicine and the Health Sciences, 111 Michigan Avenue, Northwest, Washington, DC 20010, USA

Keywords

• Timing of female puberty • Early puberty • Central precocious puberty
• Predicted adult height • Gonadotropin-releasing hormone analogues

Key points

- It is important to distinguish between common normal variations of early puberty, such as premature adrenarche and thelarche, and central precocious puberty (CPP), which may require treatment.
- A progressive increase in breast development over a 6-month period in a girl less than 8 years old, especially if accompanied by rapid growth, are the key signs suggestive of CPP.
- Treatment with gonadotropin-releasing hormone analogues, while effective in arresting puberty, is expensive, often does not improve adult height, and is being widely overused.
- Parents should be reassured that most girls with onset of puberty between age 7 and 9 do fine with monitoring and reassurance.

INTRODUCTION

Signs of early puberty are a common cause of concern among parents of children ages 5 to 9, especially in girls. In previous articles published in 2004 and 2011, the focus was on the trend for earlier puberty in girls and what might be causing it, and the benign normal variations, which are often confused with true central precocious puberty (CPP) but do not require treatment [1,2]. This review focuses on when to suspect CPP in a patient, how pediatric endocrinologists make this diagnosis, and how to target treatment with gonadotropin-releasing hormone analogues (GnRHa) to those children who are most likely to benefit.

E-mail address: pkaplowi@childrensnational.org

https://doi.org/10.1016/j.yapd.2020.04.003

WHAT HORMONES ARE INVOLVED IN PUBERTAL DEVELOPMENT?

During childhood, levels of the pituitary hormones regulating gonadal function (luteinizing hormone [LH] and follicle-stimulating hormone [FSH]) are low but begin to increase in a pulsatile fashion during early puberty, driven by the pulsatile secretion of the hypothalamic peptide gonadotropin-releasing hormone (GnRH). Rising LH stimulates the ovaries to secrete estradiol or the testes to produce testosterone, and rising FSH causes gonadal enlargement and oocyte or sperm development. Estradiol stimulates breast development and the growth spurt in females, and testosterone causes penile growth and the growth spurt in males. Pubic and axillary hair development is mainly caused by the rise in secretion of weak androgens (mainly dehydroepiandrosterone [DHEA] and its storage form DHEA-sulfate), which is independent of LH and FSH, can occur earlier than other signs of puberty, and is not a reliable indicator of CPP.

IMPORTANT BENIGN EARLY SIGNS OF PUBERTY

When a child with signs of early puberty is seen in the primary care setting, consideration of the age of the child, review of the growth chart, and a careful physical examination are critical. Age is critical because in a 1- to 3-year-old girl, breast development that progresses little over time is not uncommon and is usually caused by premature thelarche. This situation typically is managed with reassurance and a follow-up visit in 4 to 6 months to make sure there is not a significant increase in breast tissue and/or a crossing of growth percentiles upward. However, premature thelarche rarely progresses to CPP. If the child has pubic and/or axillary hair and often an adult-type body odor but no breast development (or just fat tissue in the breast area), the diagnosis is usually premature adrenarche. This is a common normal variation in pubertal development because of an early increase in the adrenal androgen DHEA. Management is parental reassurance without a need for extensive testing or treatment. Pubic hair along the labia or scrotum that appears in the first year of life with an otherwise normal examination is typically benign, although a visit to an endocrinologist may reassure the family. If an overweight girl seems to have breast tissue when sitting up that largely disappears in the supine position and no firm tissue is felt under the nipple, the child most likely has lipomastia. In some cases, follow-up observation may be needed to confirm the enlargement is not progressing. These normal variations are discussed in more detail elsewhere [2,3].

WHEN SHOULD CENTRAL PRECOCIOUS PUBERTY BE SUSPECTED AND WHAT TYPE OF EVALUATION IS NEEDED?

The key findings that suggest CPP are progressive breast development over a period of 4 to 6 months or more, accompanied by rapid growth (>6–7 cm/y), especially in girls between the ages of 6 and 8 when CPP is most common. In boys, in whom CPP is less common, progressive enlargement of both the penis and testes before age 9 is suggestive (enlargement of the penis and pubic hair without testicular enlargement or with a testicular mass is worrisome, and prompt evaluation for an adrenal or gonadal tumor or congenital adrenal hyperplasia is needed). A family history of early puberty should be sought, that is, the mother or a sister starting menses by age 10 or a father who recalls an early growth spurt relative to his peers. Also, a history of a central nervous system disorder, such as hydrocephalus, hypoxic-ischemic encephalopathy, or a brain tumor, should be noted because these conditions are associated with CPP.

Extensive hormonal testing in a child with suspected CPP can in most cases be done after the child is evaluated by a pediatric endocrinologist. However, when the previously mentioned factors are present and the specialist visit is delayed for several months, the primary care provider may proceed with ordering an LH, FSH, and either an estradiol or testosterone. A random LH $\geq$ 0.3 IU/L is considered diagnostic of CPP [4] but lower levels in the less than 0.1 to 0.2 range do not rule out the diagnosis, and a GnRH stimulation test done by the endocrinologist may be needed to confirm the diagnosis. A measurable estradiol or a testosterone of greater than 30 ng/dL support but do not prove a diagnosis of CPP. However, high levels of either estradiol or testosterone with low or undetectable LH and FSH may point to a rare case of gonadotropin-independent precocious puberty, possibly caused by a gonadal tumor. Such cases warrant prompt referral to a pediatric endocrinologist. Although many authors recommend concomitant thyroid testing, cases of CPP caused by severe hypothyroidism are extremely rare and can usually be suspected based on slow growth rate and signs and symptoms of hypothyroidism including puffy facies.

A bone age is usually done when CPP is suspected, because an advance of 2 or more years supports the diagnosis. However, since pediatric endocrinologists prefer to read bone age X-rays themselves rather than relying on the reading of an outside radiologist, it is fine to defer ordering a bone age. A bone age advanced by 2 or more years is also common in children with pubic hair only (usually premature adrenarche) and rarely indicates serious pathology [5]. Brain MRIs are often done as part of the CPP evaluation to rule out a tumor, such as a glioma or astrocytoma, or a benign developmental defect called a hypothalamic hamartoma. However, recent studies have shown that although incidental findings (pituitary microadenomas, type 1 Chiari malformations) are occasionally found, tumors or hamartomas associated with CPP are rare in 6- to 8-year-old girls [6]. Thus many endocrinologists only order brain MRIs in girls younger than age 6 and in boys, or in children with neurologic symptoms, such as frequent headaches or seizures [7].

TREATING CENTRAL PRECOCIOUS PUBERTY

GnRHa are modified preparations of the hypothalamic-releasing factor GnRH, which are designed to increase the potency and half-life of GnRH. These analogues work to block puberty because they have a sustained action on the receptors for GnRH in the pituitary, which require pulsatile exposure to native GnRH. They were initially developed to treat prostate cancer by lowering testosterone secretion, which the tumor cells require. In 1986, the first long-term study of daily GnRHa treatment of CPP in 27 children treated for 2 to 4 years showed that GnRHa treatment clearly slowed growth velocity and skeletal maturation, while improving predicted adult height (PAH) based on bone age [8,9]. In that study the mean age at treatment initiation (5.2 years), growth rate (10.9 cm/y), bone age advancement (>3 years), estradiol in girls (42 pg/mL) and testosterone in boys (471 ng/dL), breast Tanner stage (3.3), and testicular volume (16 mL) indicate that this cohort was much younger and progressing more rapidly than most children with CPP treated today. In 1993 the Food and Drug Administration approved the monthly version of a GnRHa (leuprolide acetate [Lupron Depot]) to treat CPP. Since then, the use of GnRHa to treat CPP has steadily increased and several additional formulations have been introduced, including a 3-month injectable forms of Lupron, and an implant called Supprelin, which releases the GnRHa histrelin for at least a year. Most recently in 2017, a 6-month GnRHa, triptorelin (Triptodur), received Food and Drug Administration approval. The advantages and disadvantages of these various forms of therapy are summarized in Table 1.

One indicator of the rapid expansion of GnRHa use in recent years are data provided by one marketer of GnRHa, showing that between 2012 and 2017, the median age of GnRHa therapy initiation in girls (which is likely on the

Table 1
Preparations of gonadotropin-releasing hormone analogues currently in use in United States

Brand name (chemical name)	Dose formulations (mg)	Frequency of administration	Advantages	Disadvantages
Lupron Depot-Ped (leuprolide)	7.5, 11.25, or 15	Monthly	Possibly more rapid onset of effect	Need for frequent injections
Lupron Depot-Ped (leuprolide)	11.25 or 30	Every 3 mo	Fewer injections than 1 mo form with similar efficacy	No less expensive than monthly
Triptodur (triptorelin)	22.5	Every 6 mo	Fewer injections than Lupron	No less expensive than 1 mo and 3 mo formulations
Supprelin (histrelin)	50	Implant is designed to last at least 12 mo	No injections; effect may last for up to 2 y	Needs to be placed and removed by a simple surgical procedure

average about 6 months after the onset of pubertal changes) was 9.0 years for Supprelin and Depot Lupron Ped [10]. Furthermore, only 11.6% of patients who had received Lupron depot and 15.1% of patients who had received Supprelin were started on treatment before age 8. These data indicate that most girls now being treated for CPP are starting puberty at the early end of the current normal range.

EVIDENCE FOR A DECLINE IN THE AGE OF PUBERTY ONSET: THE REASON FOR MORE TREATMENT?

During the 1960s to 1970s the mean age of onset of breast development (thelarche) was 10.5 to 11 years, but data from the 1990s and later suggest a significant decline in the mean age of thelarche, with a smaller decline in the mean age of menarche. In a landmark study of more than 17,000 girls (ages 3–12 years) screened in physicians' offices around the country [11] the mean age of onset of breast development was 8.9 years for African-American and 10.0 years for white girls. Furthermore, 5% of white 7 to 8 year olds and 15.4% of African-American 7 to 8 year old girls already had breast development on examination. More recently, in nearly 1000 girls of 7 to 8 years old, 10% of white, 23% of African-American, and 15% of Hispanic girls had reached at least Tanner 2 breast development [12]. There is mounting evidence that the trend for increasing obesity is a major driver of this trend [13]. Consequently, continued adherence to prior definitions for precocious puberty (breast development before 8 years of age) has resulted in an increasing proportion of girls being categorized as precocious. In response to this secular trend of earlier puberty, guidelines were proposed in 1999 recommending that precocious puberty be redefined as onset of breast development before 7 years for white girls and before 6 years for African-American girls [14]. However, the traditional definition of female precocious puberty (ie, starting before age 8 years) is still what most primary care providers adhere to in deciding which patients to refer for further evaluation.

Ambiguity in the diagnostic criteria for sexual precocity has provided a fertile environment for an increase in treatment of borderline CPP cases (ie, with pubertal onset between 7 and 9 years of age). Availability of treatment itself can encourage "medicalization" of physiologic variations of normal development as pathologic disorders in need of therapy. Justification of treatment often relies on assumptions about morbidity (eg, psychological distress) or undesired outcomes (eg, reduced adult height) that seem reasonable but, in fact, are not well documented. In these situations, it is challenging to discern if GnRHa therapy for early puberty is a medically necessary intervention for which the benefit justifies its cost burden on the patient and family.

After approval of monthly Lupron Depot, one expert proposed that treatment be limited to patients with complete and progressive CPP with pubertal hormone concentrations, plus abnormal height potential, which refers to a

PAH, based on current height and bone age, of less than fifth percentile, or psychosocial morbidity/distress (eg, early menses in mentally or emotionally immature individuals) [15]. Another commentary urged caution in starting treatment before it is clear that puberty is progressing rapidly [16].

The following case scenario illustrates different factors that influence the decision to initiate pubertal suppression. These factors are then critically evaluated for available evidence supporting prescribing, or withholding, GnRHa therapy.

An 8-year-old white girl was noted to have breast development and pubic hair by her parents at age 7 years 9 months. The family history is negative for early puberty. The parents are of average height (the girl's target height is 5 ft, 4 in or 162.5 cm based on parental height). Growth earlier in childhood had been along the 75th percentile in height and 90th percentile in weight, but is now at the 90th to 95th percentile (137 cm) in height and the 95th percentile in weight. The examination reveals Tanner stage 2 breast development (2 cm of glandular breast tissue bilaterally) and pubic hair. Bone age is 10 years, yielding a PAH of 164 cm (5 ft, 4.5 in). The child is in third grade and has no apparent emotional issues. Her parents request treatment to suppress puberty because they were told by the pediatrician that without treatment she would stop growing early and end up short, and they are not ready for her to start her menstrual cycles.

DO GONADOTROPIN-RELEASING HORMONE ANALOGUES INCREASE ADULT HEIGHT IN CHILDREN WITH CENTRAL PRECOCIOUS PUBERTY?

The primary rationale for medical suppression of CPP is concern that growth plates will fuse prematurely resulting in height attainment significantly lower than genetic target height. Indeed, treatment of children with very early onset of CPP often results in an adult height that significantly exceeds PAH at initiation of therapy. In one study of girls who started treatment before age 5 years, the adult height (164.6 cm) far exceeded the mean adult height of a separate group of untreated females (152.5 cm). However, for patients started on treatment after age 5 years, the results were much less impressive (mean adult height of 157.6 cm) [17]. This dependence of increased height on younger age of GnRHa treatment initiation has been found in other studies. In 46 Italian girls with onset of puberty between 7.5 and 8.5 years either treated with monthly GnRHa or not treated, the mean adult heights were similar (158–159 cm) in the treated and untreated groups, and not significantly different from the midparental height (MPH) [18]. In a study from Israel of 22 girls diagnosed before age 6 years and 38 girls diagnosed between ages 6 and 8 years, both groups had a similar mean PAH (152.8 cm to 154.6 cm) before onset of therapy. Those starting treatment before 6 years had a mean adult height of 162.8 cm, which actually exceeded their parental MPH of 159.3 cm. The patients with treatment onset at 6 to 8 years had a mean adult height of 157.9 cm, equal to their MPH [19]. Recently, a meta-analysis of GnRH therapy for girls with onset of puberty in the low end of the normal range (8–9 years) showed no overall difference in adult height versus girls allowed to go through puberty spontaneously [20].

In response to the uncertainty regarding the growth benefit of GnRHa therapy in CPP, a consensus statement by the North American and European Pediatric Endocrine Societies made the following recommendations:

- "The greatest height gain has been observed in girls with onset of puberty at less than 6 years (average height gain 9–10 cm). Girls with onset between 6 and 8 comprise a heterogeneous group that may have a moderate benefit ranging from 4.5 to 7.2 cm. *The decision to initiate therapy in girls with onset after age 6 should be individualized.*" [21]
- "Progressive pubertal development and growth acceleration should be documented over a 3 to 6 month period before GnRH therapy" [21]. This was included because some girls display a slowly progressive form of CPP and achieve adult heights within their target range without intervention [22,23].

Perhaps a more relevant question to address in justifying GnRHa treatment is how often girls with untreated CPP fail to reach a normal adult height. In one report of 20 girls initially evaluated at a mean age of 7 years after a mean onset of breast tissue at 5.6 years, mean adult height was normal at 161.4 cm, and 90% achieved a normal adult height of more than 153 cm [24]. A more recent but larger study from Thailand followed 104 girls with breast development starting between the ages of 7.0 and 9.0 until near-final height. Although the average age at menarche was also early at 10.2 years, the near final height was 154.0 cm, which was similar to the MPH of 153.1 cm [25]. Unfortunately, there are few other studies examining this question, likely caused by evolution of standard practice in recent years to treat rather than monitor girls with CPP. Based on the literature and personal experience, most girls evaluated for CPP after age 6 years have a PAH within the normal adult range (ie, 5 ft, 1 in, or 155 cm or greater). Thus, justification for treating girls with mildly early CPP is usually not to avoid an abnormally short adult height, but rather to address parental concerns about differences in family expectations for height or anticipated psychological harm.

DO GIRLS WITH CENTRAL PRECOCIOUS PUBERTY HAVE MORE PSYCHOLOGICAL PROBLEMS THAN PREPUBERTAL GIRLS THEIR AGE?

There is a common belief that girls with CPP have a higher incidence of behavioral problems than prepubertal girls of similar age. In one early often-cited study, 9 of 33 girls (27%) with CPP who took the Child Behavior Checklist scored greater than or equal to two standard deviations higher than the mean on the total behavior problem scale and 48% scored greater than two standard deviations higher than the mean on the social withdrawal scale. The authors concluded that although "elevated sex steroid levels might contribute to increased aggressive and hyperactive behaviors, they may be modified by social and environmental factors" [26]. In one of the few studies that looked at behavioral changes during CPP treatment, 20 girls with CPP expressed concerns about physical differences from their peers at baseline. Fifteen girls who were followed during treatment felt less embarrassed about pubertal development as breast tissue regressed. However, elevated scores of withdrawal, anxiety/depression, and somatic complaints persisted [27].

Another study of 36 girls with signs of early puberty included 15 patients with CPP, 8 with premature adrenarche, and 13 had early normal puberty. All girls with CPP were treated with GnRHa. Baseline psychological assessments of cognitive competence, peer acceptance, physical competence, and maternal acceptance were, on average, normal in all groups. After 1 year of follow-up, findings were "largely reassuring regarding concerns of adverse physical consequences of early puberty in girls" [28]. Another study of 15 girls with CPP and 15 age-matched control subjects concluded that treated CPP girls did not differ in their cognitive or psychological functioning from control girls [29]. In summary, with few studies using different patient selection criteria and reporting different prevalence of behavioral problems in CPP girls, it remains unclear if psychosocial stress should be considered a predictable consequence of early puberty. Thus, it is debatable that potential stress should be factored into making a decision to start GnRHa therapy, and it is not established that such treatment alleviates stress.

IS PREVENTION OF POTENTIAL EARLY MENARCHE IN GIRLS WITH CENTRAL PRECOCIOUS PUBERTY NECESSARY?

Parents who request treatment of girls with CPP often fear their daughter will not be able to handle the stress of experiencing and caring for early menses. However, when puberty starts at age 7.5 to 8 years and is not suppressed, menarche usually does not occur until age 10 or later, because it typically takes 2 to 3 years to progress from thelarche to menarche [30]. How strong is the evidence that girls having menarche close to 10 years of age experience significant distress and, if so, benefit from GnRHa treatment designed to delay menarche until age 11 years or later? There are no studies that directly address this question in a controlled setting. It is understandable that anxiety associated with early menses is often experienced by mothers. It also seems reasonable that a girl prepared for early menses by a calm and reassuring parent or guardian may handle it better. However, in the absence of data and in the presence of so much individual family variation on this issue, counseling parents who desire treatment to delay menses remains challenging. One suggestion could be to point out that (1) many early maturing girls progress slowly and do not have menarche before age 10 years, (2) most girls having menarche between the ages of 9 and 10 adjust to having menstrual periods well after the first couple of cycles, and (3) if menses do start early and are deemed too stressful, initiation of GnRHa could still promptly suppress subsequent menses. Alternatively, the child could be started on medroxyprogesterone (Depo-Provera) to reduce the amount and frequency of bleeding at a minimal cost. This option is especially relevant for the care of children with developmental disabilities, in whom treatment solely to suppress menses may alleviate significant distress for patients and care providers [31].

HOW LONG SHOULD TREATMENT OF CENTRAL PRECOCIOUS PUBERTY WITH GONADOTROPIN-RELEASING HORMONE ANALOGUES CONTINUE?

To return to our previous case

The parents express a strong desire to treat their daughter to delay the onset of menses. She is started on Lupron Depot Ped, 11.25 mg given intramuscularly every 3 months. At her next visit 4 months later, she is growing at a normal rate and the breast tissue has regressed. Treatment is planned to continue until age 10 years. However, a year later, when she is 9.75 years old and receiving her last scheduled dose of GnRHa, the parents ask to continue treatment for another year because they are concerned that their child is too emotionally fragile to handle menses. Based on the latest bone age her PAH is 5 ft, 5 in.

There are no widely accepted guidelines for how long to continue treatment with a GnRHa for CPP and individual practice varies widely. The consensus statement on the use of GnRHa lists "maximizing height, synchronizing puberty with peers, ameliorating psychological distress, and facilitating care of the developmentally delayed child" as factors to consider [21]. In the studies reviewed, the mean age of treatment discontinuation varied from 10.6 to 12 years, with mean bone age at discontinuation ranging from 12.1 to 13.9 years and mean age of menarche at 12.3 years [21]. An important question for those girls whose treatment is based on the desire to delay menarche, is whether the targeted age at menarche should be closer to 10, 11, or 12 years, or to what extent parents should have the final say on when their child should be allowed to reach menarche. On average menarche occurs about 1 year (range, 6–18 months) after discontinuation of GnRHa therapy. Stopping treatment by age 10 years should ensure menarche does not occur until age 10.5 to 11.5 years, which is considered to be in the lower part of the normal range. It is difficult to defend an expectation for insurance companies or public funds to continue to pay $20,000 to 40,000 per year for GnRHa to delay menarche until age 12 years or later, which is close to the population average. Consequently, it seems reasonable to discontinue GnRHa no later than 10 years in most cases. At that age, resumption of thelarche is close to the current population average and suppression of menses by other much lower cost measures, such as Depo-Provera, is available and effective if needed.

Treatment decisions with GnRHa therapies, like all medical interventions, should attempt to balance benefits, risks, and costs for the individual child. Toward this goal, the following should be included in an informed discussion when GnRHa treatment is being considered for an early maturing girl (eg, 6–8 years of age) [32]:

1. Your child's adult height, especially if she is taller than average now, will probably be normal and may not significantly increase after treatment
2. It is uncertain whether your child will experience adverse psychosocial stress from early puberty or, if she does, whether GnRHa treatment would prevent or alleviate such stress

3. Your child may have slow progression of puberty so that menstrual periods may not occur as early as feared
4. It is not necessary to prevent a first menstrual period to intervene and stop subsequent menses
5. Costs of treatment are high (currently in the range of $20,000–40,000 per year) and need to be added to the costs and stress of frequent follow-up clinic visits and periodic injections or having an implant placed

Such a discussion encourages thoughtful consideration of therapeutic restraint, reassurance, and observation of many girls who might otherwise receive 2 to 4 years of treatment for a poorly defined benefit achieved at a high cost.

SUMMARY

Although many children, especially girls, are evaluated for signs of early puberty, only a small proportion have CPP, which is the only form that benefits from medical therapy. The most reliable indicator in girls is progressive breast enlargement before age 8 accompanied by rapid growth in height. Even for girls whose diagnosis of CPP is confirmed by a specialist, treatment may not be necessary. Studies show that girls whose onset of puberty is at age 7 or later usually achieve normal height and that treatment with GnRHa may not result in improvement in adult height. Although early onset of puberty and menses may be stressful for some children and their parents, counseling and reassurance may be helpful in decreasing the overuse of this effective but expensive therapy.

Disclosure

The author has nothing to disclose.

References

[1] Kaplowitz PB. Precocious puberty: update on secular trends, diagnosis, testing, and treatment. Adv Pediatr 2004;51:37–62.
[2] Kaplowitz PB. Update on precocious puberty: girls are showing signs of puberty earlier but most do not require treatment. Adv Pediatr 2011;58:243–58.
[3] Kaplowitz P, Bloch C, the Section On Endocrinology. Clinical report: evaluation and referral of children with signs of early puberty. Pediatrics 2016;137(1):e20153732.
[4] Houk CP, Kunselman AR, Lee PA. Adequacy of a single unstimulated luteinizing hormone level to diagnose central precocious puberty in girls. Pediatrics 2009;123(6):e1059–63.
[5] Desalvo D, Vaidyanathan P, Mehra R, et al. In children with premature adrenarche, bone age advancement by 2 or more years is common and generally benign. J Pediatr Endocrinol Metab 2013;26:215–21.
[6] Pedicelli S, Alessio P, Scire G, et al. Routine screening by brain magnetic resonance imaging is not indicated in every girl with onset of puberty between ages of 6 and 8. J Clin Endocrinol Metab 2014;99:4455–61.
[7] Kaplowitz PB. Do 6-8 year old girls with central precocious puberty need routine brain imaging? Int J Pediatr Endocrinol 2016;2016:9.
[8] Pescovitz OH, Comite F, Hench K, et al. The NIH experience with precocious puberty: diagnostic subgroups and response to short-term luteinizing hormone releasing hormone analogue therapy. J Pediatr 1986;108:47–54.

[9] Comite F, Cassorla F, Barnes K, et al. Luteinizing hormone releasing hormone analogue therapy for central precocious puberty: long-term effect on somatic growth, bone maturation, and predicted height. JAMA 1986;255:2613–6.
[10] Grubb E, Dragnic S. AbbVie data in file. 2018.
[11] Herman-Giddens ME, Slora EJ, Wasserman RC, et al. Secondary sexual characteristics and menses in young girls seen in office practice: a study from the Pediatric Research in Office Settings network. Pediatrics 1997;99:505–12.
[12] Biro FM, Galvez MP, Greenspan LC, et al. Pubertal assessment method and baseline characteristics in a mixed longitudinal study of girls. Pediatrics 2010;126:e583–90.
[13] Biro FM, Greenspan LC, Galvez MP. Puberty in girls of the 21st century. J Pediatr Adolesc Gynecol 2012;25:289–94.
[14] Kaplowitz PB, Oberfield SE. Reexamination of the age limit for defining when puberty is precocious in girls in the United States: implications for evaluation and treatment. Pediatrics 1999;104:936–41.
[15] Rosenfield RL. Selection of children with precocious puberty for treatment with gonadotropin releasing hormone analogs. J Pediatr 1994;124:989–91.
[16] Klein KO. Editorial: precocious puberty. Who has it? Who should be treated? J Clin Endocrinol Metab 1999;84:411–4.
[17] Paul D, Conte F, Grumbach MM, et al. Long-term effect of gonadotropin-releasing hormone agonist therapy on final and near-final height in 26 children with true precocious puberty treated at a median age of less than 5 years. J Clin Endocrinol Metab 1995;80:546–51.
[18] Cassio A, Cacciari E, Balsamo A, et al. Randomized trial of LHRH analogue treatment on final height in girls with onset of puberty aged 7.5-8.5 years. Arch Dis Child 1999;81: 329–32.
[19] Lazar L, Padoa A, Phillip M. Growth pattern and final height after cessation of gonadotropin-suppressive therapy in girls with central sexual precocity. J Clin Endocrinol Metab 2007;92: 483–9.
[20] Bertelloni S, Massart F, Miccoli M, et al. Adult height after spontaneous pubertal growth or GnRH analog treatment in girls with early puberty: a meta-analysis. Eur J Pedaitr 2017;176: 697–704.
[21] Carel JC, Eugster EA, Rogol A, et al. Consensus statement on the use of gonadotropin-releasing hormone analogs in children. Pediatrics 2009;123:e752–62.
[22] Palmert MR, Malin HV, Boepple PA. Unsustained or slowly progressive puberty in young girls: Initial presentation and long-term follow-up of 20 untreated patients. J Clin Endocrinol Metab 1999;84:415–23.
[23] Masset F, Federico G, Harrell JC, et al. Growth outcomes during GnRH agonist treatments for slowly-progressive central precocious puberty. Neuroendocrinology 2009;90:307–14.
[24] Bar A, Linder B, Sobel EH, et al. Bayley-Pinneau method of height prediction in girls with central precocious puberty: correlation with adult height. J Pediatr 1995;126:955–8.
[25] Jaruratanasirikul S, Thongkum K, Krisaneepaiboon S, et al. Girls with early puberty attain a near-final height similar to their target height. J Pediatr Endocrinol Metab 2011;24: 339–45.
[26] Sonis WA, Comite F, Blue J, et al. Behavior problems and social competence in girls with true precocious puberty. J Pediatr 1985;106:156–60.
[27] Xhrouet-Heinrichs D, Lagrou K, Heinrichs C, et al. Longitudinal study of behavioral and affective patterns in girls with central precocious puberty during long-acting triptorelin therapy. Acta Paediatr 1997;86:808–15.
[28] Schoelwer MJ, Donahue KL, Diddrick P, et al. One-year follow-up of girls with precocious puberty and their mothers: do psychological assessments change over time or with treatment? Horm Res Paediatr 2017;88:347–53.
[29] Wojniusz S, Callens N, Sutterlin S, et al. Cognitive, emotional, and psychosocial functioning of girls treated with pharmacological blockage for idiopathic central precocious puberty. Front Psychol 2016;7:1–12.

[30] Biro FM, Huang B, Crawford PB, et al. Pubertal correlates in black and white girls. J Pediatr 2006;148(2):234–40.
[31] Albanese A, Hopper NW. Suppression of menstruation in adolescents with severe learning disabilities. Arch Dis Child 2007;92:629–32.
[32] Kaplowitz PB, Backeljauw PF, Allen DB. Toward more targeted and cost-effective gonadotropin-releasing hormone analog treatment in girls with central precocious puberty. Horm Res Paediatr 2018;90:1–7.

Advances in Pediatrics 67 (2020) 105–112
ADVANCES IN PEDIATRICS

Urolithiasis in Children

Valerie Panzarino, MD
Department of Pediatrics, University of South Florida, 17 Davis Boulevard, Suite 200, Tampa, FL 33606, USA

Keywords
• Urolithiasis • Nephrolithiasis • Kidney stones • Children

Key points

- Ultrasonography of the urinary tract not renal computed tomography scan should be the primary initial imaging tool used in the evaluation of pediatric urolithiasis.
- All pediatric patients with urolithiasis should undergo urinary metabolic evaluation secondary to the increased incidence of associated metabolic abnormalities and subsequent high risk of stone recurrence.
- Calcium-containing stones are the most frequent stones in children. Decreased urine volume, increased urinary supersaturation of calcium oxalate and calcium phosphate, hypercalciuria, and hypocitraturia are predisposing factors.
- Treatment of pediatric urolithiasis includes dietary, medical, and surgical interventions, which vary depending on the size, location, and type of stone and underlying urinary metabolic abnormality.

INTRODUCTION

Pediatric urolithiasis is increasing, with an associated increase in medical cost [1–3]. A study published in 2015 estimated the cost of pediatric urolithiasis in the United States to be $146 million per year for emergency department care and $229 million per year for hospitalization [3]. The incidence and specific risk factors (Box 1) vary based on region, race, gender, socioeconomic status, and dietary habits [4–6].

A recent pediatric study using a large insurance claim database in the United States reported a peak incidence of pediatric urolithiasis of 65.2 cases per 100,000 person-years [5]. In South Carolina, a study reported a pronounced increase in stones in adolescent girls in particular, with a 57% higher incidence of stones in girls age 15 to 19 years compared with boys of the same age [7].

E-mail address: vpanzari@usf.edu

https://doi.org/10.1016/j.yapd.2020.03.004
0065-3101/20/

Box 1: Risk factors for pediatric urolithiasis

- Female gender, more than 10 years of age
- Non-Hispanic white race
- South east region of the United States
- Increasing age
- Underlying genitourinary abnormality

Emergency department visits and hospitalizations for pediatric urolithiasis have also increased; 1 study showed an increase from 0.048% for all emergency department visits in 1999 to 0.089% for all emergency department visits in 2008, which was an 86% increase [8]. Understanding stone formation risk factors, evaluation, and treatment options is essential to the care of pediatric patients with urolithiasis.

CLINICAL PRESENTATION

The clinical presentation and stone composition in pediatric patients with urolithiasis vary based on several factors: age, sex, dietary intake, time period, and geographic region. Abdominal pain and flank pain are the most common presenting symptoms. In 1 single-center study from a North American tertiary care center, flank pain occurred in 63% of pediatric patients with stones, with 82% discovered to have microscopic hematuria during the evaluation [6]. Other potential presenting symptoms are dysuria, gross hematuria, urgency, nausea, and vomiting. The classic description of excruciating loin pain associated with the passage of a stone usually seen in adults is not typically seen in children [9,10]. In infants, stone pain can easily be mistaken for colic and gastrointestinal causes of abdominal pain. Younger children tend to present with a greater stone burden and have primarily renal stones, whereas older children tend to have ureteral stones and have higher spontaneous stone passage rates [11,12]. One study of 102 very-low-birth-weight infants showed that 6% had renal calcification discovered as an incidental finding [13].

The formation of urinary tract stones is a complicated process depending on the interplay between multiple factors (Box 2) [10].

Box 2: Factors influencing stone formation

- Urine pH
- Urine concentration of stone-forming metabolites
- Urine volume
- Balance between crystallization-promoting and crystallization-inhibiting factors
- Anatomic abnormalities causing urinary stasis
- Presence of foreign bodies

The most common type of stone in children is calcium oxalate, accounting for 45% to 65% of the stones [14–16]. Struvite or magnesium ammonium phosphate stones account for 3% to 30% of stones in children, with a higher incidence in Europe and developing countries than in North America, and may have a staghorn shape if they are formed in the renal calyx. Struvite stones are typically associated with urinary tract infections secondary to urease-splitting organisms that generate ammonium and bicarbonate, such as *Proteus*, and may be associated with an increased urine pH. In the United States, struvite stones are most often seen in children with abnormalities of the urogenital tract that predispose them to urinary tract infection, such as horseshoe kidney or neurogenic bladder requiring intermittent catheterization [12]. Other stones, including cystine and uric acid stones, account for only 5% to 10% of stones in children [14–16] (Box 3).

EVALUATION

The evaluation of possible pediatric urolithiasis should begin with a thorough history and physical examination. The history should include the presence or absence of abnormalities of the urinary tract; urinary tract infection; prematurity; family history of kidney stones; ketogenic diet; malabsorption; medications associated with stone formation; immobilization; and dietary excesses of calcium, phosphorus, or sodium.

Further evaluation should include urinalysis with microscopic evaluation, followed by a urine culture if indicated, and imaging of the urinary tract (Box 4). Plain abdominal radiographs of the kidneys, ureter, and bladder (KUB) alone have low sensitivity (62%) and specificity (67%) for stone disease [17]. Although renal computed tomography (CT) scan is a commonly used imaging modality in adults, it should be avoided in the initial evaluation of pediatric urolithiasis because of the potential cumulative effects of radiation. In children, the sensitivity and specificity of renal ultrasonography and a KUB approaches that of a renal CT scan, although small and distal ureteral stones could be missed on renal ultrasonography. Studies showed that the presence of those small stones did not alter the management of the patients and were therefore not clinically significant [18,19].

Once kidney stones are confirmed, further evaluation should include a basic metabolic panel to screen for acidosis; evaluation of serum electrolytes and calcium levels; blood urea nitrogen and creatinine levels; and serum phosphorous,

Box 3: Pediatric stone composition

- Calcium-containing stones are the most common type in children
- Struvite stones are more common in developing countries; in the United States they are often associated with underlying genitourinary abnormalities
- Cystine and uric acid stones are uncommon and are associated with underlying metabolic stone-forming disorders

Box 4: Urinary tract imaging in pediatric urolithiasis

- Urinary tract ultrasonography should be the primary initial imaging modality for evaluation of possible urolithiasis in children, not renal computed tomography.

magnesium, and uric acid levels. Additional studies may include a 25-hydroxyvitamin D level and parathyroid hormone level to further investigate calcium and phosphorus metabolism. The urine should be strained in an effort to catch the stone so that it can be sent for stone analysis. Urinary metabolic evaluation should be postponed until the acute event has resolved and stone fragments are no longer being passed. The 24-hour urine collection for metabolic evaluation should include total urine volume, sodium, potassium, calcium, magnesium, oxalate, uric acid, cystine screen, citrate, phosphorus, pH, and creatinine, and calculation of the supersaturations of calcium oxalate, calcium phosphate, and uric acid.

An underlying urinary metabolic abnormality can be identified in more than 50% of children with urolithiasis and these children have a 38% to 50% chance of stone recurrence [11,20–22]. Children 10 years old or younger have the highest rate of recurrence, whereas children without an identified underlying metabolic disorder have a less than 10% chance of recurrence [11]. A study from South Carolina by Sas and colleagues [23] of 155 children with stone disease showed that the most commonly identified 24-hour urine abnormalities were low urine volumes, increased supersaturation of calcium oxalate and calcium phosphate, and hypercalciuria. Other studies identify hypocitraturia and hypercalciuria as the most common urinary metabolic abnormalities [24].

TREATMENT

Once a kidney stone is diagnosed, hydration should be encouraged in all patients in order to decrease urinary supersaturation. One goal is for children to drink 1000 mL/1.73 m^2/d; however, fluid goals are rarely achieved [25]. One intervention to improve adherence with the hydration prescription is to tell school-aged children that "dilution is the solution to pollution" and provide them a note for school allowing a water bottle and frequent bathroom breaks. Foods high in oxalate should be limited, including ice tea, rhubarb, grits, okra, peanuts, and chocolate. Certain fruits and vegetables are high in potassium and increase urinary citrate levels, thus providing protection against stone formation [26]. A low-sodium or no-added-sodium diet should be instituted because it has been shown to decrease urinary calcium level [27–29] but calcium intake must not be restricted. A diet high in calcium has been shown to decrease stone formation in adults [30]. Sodium intake should be limited to less than 2 to 3 mEq/kg/d for young children or less than 2.4 g in adolescents or adults [31]. In addition, dark sodas containing high phosphate levels should be avoided. In adults, animal protein restriction decreases calcium oxalate production [32], but protein should not be restricted in children during periods of growth.

In addition to general dietary changes, specific dietary and medical intervention is indicated if an underlying metabolic disorder is identified (Table 1). Hypocitraturia is a common urinary metabolic abnormality in children with stones. It can be seen in patients with the complete form of distal renal tubular acidosis [33]. For adults with hypocitraturia, increased intake of lemonade has been shown to reduce stone recurrence in some studies, but not all [34]. Hypocitraturia in children can be successfully treated with potassium citrate supplementation [35].

Hypercalciuria is also common in children with urolithiasis and is associated with increased urinary sodium excretion. A genetic predisposition and abnormalities in vitamin D metabolism have also been suggested. Specific treatment targets decreasing urinary sodium and urinary calcium excretion and includes salt restriction and thiazide diuretics if needed [35,36]. Potassium citrate therapy may further reduce stone formation in patients with hypercalciuria.

Hyperoxaluria predisposes to stone formation. Primary hyperoxaluria is a rare autosomal recessive genetic disorder with 3 main types. The severity can range from recurrent stone formation to the development of oxalosis, which is the systemic deposition of oxalate with renal failure. Primary hyperoxaluria type 1 is the most frequent type and is caused by low or absent liver-specific peroxisomal alanine glyoxylate aminotransferase (AGT) level. Diagnosis is based on genetic sequencing. Infants who present with hyperoxaluria are severely affected [37,38]. Secondary hyperoxaluria caused by increased intestinal oxalate absorption can occur in children with malabsorption or chronic inflammatory bowel disease [39]. Initial treatment includes hydration and oxalate-restricted diet, even though only 10% of urinary oxalate is derived from nutritional intake [37]. The rest is endogenously produced in the liver. Treatment with potassium citrate, magnesium, and pyrophosphates is used to decrease stone formation. Targeted therapy with pyridoxine to decrease oxalate production in the liver can be helpful in patients with primary

Table 1
Specific treatment of urinary metabolic abnormalities

Disorder	Treatment options
Hypocitraturia	Increased dietary potassium and possibly citrate Potassium citrate supplementation
Hypercalciuria	Dietary salt restriction No dietary calcium restriction Thiazide diuretics
Hyperoxaluria	Dietary oxalate restriction Trial of pyridoxine in primary hyperoxaluria Potassium citrate, magnesium, and pyrophosphate supplementation
Cystinuria	Potassium citrate supplementation Tiopronin
Hyperuricosuria	Potassium citrate supplementation Allopurinol, especially if increased serum uric acid levels

hyperoxaluria type 1 [40]. In severe forms in which renal failure develops, a liver-kidney combined transplant is optimal so that the transplant kidney is not at risk for stone recurrence.

Cystinuria is another rare autosomal recessive disorder associated with recurrent stones caused by mutations in genes that control reabsorption of certain amino acids, including cystine. Measures to decrease stone recurrence in cystinuria include citrate therapy and hydration to decrease stone formation, in addition to an agent to decrease cystine excretion in the urine, such as tiopronin. Tiopronin has been approved by the US Food and Drug Administration as an orphan product to treat this condition [41,42].

Uric acid stones are radio-opaque and account for 2% to 4% of urolithiasis in children [14,16]. They are seen in patients with hyperuricosuria and an acidic urine pH; myelodysplasia; metabolic disorders with increased serum uric acid levels, such as Lesch-Nyhan syndrome; and in pediatric patients on the ketogenic diet [43]. They may require treatment with allopurinol to normalize serum uric acid levels and potassium citrate to decrease stone formation.

UROLOGIC INTERVENTION

The acute care of children with symptomatic stones should include hydration and appropriate analgesia, nonsteroidal antiinflammatory drugs, acetaminophen, and short-term opiate agonists. Ward and colleagues [5] reported the use of opiate agonists in 40% of pediatric patients with urolithiasis. Pediatric urology consultation should be obtained in all children with suspected urinary tract obstruction secondary to urolithiasis. Urologic surgery is necessary in 25% to 50% of pediatric patients with urolithiasis [44,45]. Surgical options include shock wave lithotripsy, retrograde intrarenal surgery with ureteroscopy, and percutaneous nephrolithotomy. Percutaneous nephrolithotomy is typically reserved for large stones or children with complicated urinary tracts, such as horseshoe kidney or reconstructed bladders [46]. Ward and colleagues [5] reported retrograde intrarenal surgery with ureteroscopy to be the most frequent intervention in children. Initial treatment should include observation with or without expulsion therapy using an α-blocker, tamsulosin, in pediatric patients with uncomplicated ureteral stones less than or equal to 10 mm [47]. Stones less than 5 mm have a high rate of spontaneous passage. Recent studies suggest that medical expulsive therapy in children with distal ureteral stones increases the rate of spontaneous stone passage and has a low incidence of adverse events [48].

SUMMARY

The management of children with urolithiasis requires a multifaceted approach including pediatric nephrology and urology expertise. Evaluation and treatment should be pediatric focused, minimizing radiation exposure and reducing risk of stone recurrence.

Disclosure

The author has nothing to disclose.

References

[1] Edvardsson VO, Ingvarsdottir SE, Palsson R, et al. Incidence of kidney stone disease in icelandic children and adolescents from 1985 to 2013: results of a nationwide study. Pediatr Nephrol 2018;33(8):1375–84.
[2] Sas DJ, Hulsy TC, Shatat IF, et al. Increasing incidence of kidney stones in children evaluated in the emergency department. J Peds 2010;157(1):132–7.
[3] Wang HH, Wiener JS, Lipkin ME, et al. Estimating the nationwide, hospital based economic impact of pediatric urolithiasis. J Urol 2015;93(5):1855–9.
[4] Clayton DB, Pope JC. The increasing pediatric stone disease problem. Ther Adv Urol 2011;3(1):3–12.
[5] Ward JB, Feinstein L, Pierce C, et al. Pediatric urinary stone disease in the United States: the urologic diseases in America project. Urol 2019;129:180.
[6] Kit LC, Filler G, Pike J, et al. Pediatric urolithiasis: experience at a tertiary care pediatric hospital. Can Urol Assoc J 2008;2(4):381–6.
[7] Tasian GE, Ross ME, Song L, et al. Annual incidence of nephrolithiasis among children and adults in South Carolina from 1997 to 2012. Clin J Am Soc Nephrol 2016;11(3):488–96.
[8] Kairam N, Allegra JR, Eskin B. Rise in emergency department visits of pediatric patients for renal colic from 1999 – 2008. Pediatr Emerg Care 2013;29(4):462–4.
[9] Routh JC, Graham DA, Nelson CP. Epidemiologic trends in pediatric urolithiasis at united states free standing pediatric hospitals. J Urol 2010;184(3):1100–4.
[10] Hutton SA. Evaluation of urinary tract calculi in children. Arch Dis Child 2001;84:320–3.
[11] Pietrow P, Pope JC, Adams MC, et al. Clinical outcome of pediatric stone disease. J Urol 2002;167(2 Pt 1):670–3.
[12] Barroso U, Jednak R, Felming P, et al. Bladder calculi in children who perform clean intermittent catheterization. BJU Int 2000;85:879.
[13] Chang HY, Chyong-Hsin H, Jeng-Daw T, et al. Renal calcification in very low birth weight infants. Pediatr Neonatol 2011;52(3):145–9.
[14] Stapleton FB. Childhood stones. Endocrinol Metab Clin North Am 2002;31:1001–15.
[15] Asplin JR. Evaluation of the kidney stone patient. Semin Nephrol 2008;28:99–110.
[16] Milliner DS, Murphy ME. Urolithiasis in pediatric patients. Mayo Clin Proc 1993;68(3):241–8.
[17] Roth CS, Bowyer BA, Berquist TH. Utility of the plain abdominal radiograph for diagnosing ureteral calculi. Ann Emerg Med 1985;14:311.
[18] Catalano O, Nunziata A, Altei F, et al. Suspected ureteral colic: primary helical CT versus selective helical CT after unenhanced radiography and sonography. AJR Am J Roentgenol 2002;178:379–87.
[19] Ripollés T, Agramunt M, Errando J, et al. Suspected ureteral colic: plain film and sonography vs unenhanced helical CT. A prospective study in 66 patients. Eur Radiol 2004;14(1):129–36.
[20] VanDervoort K, Wiesen J, Frank R, et al. Urolithiasis in pediatric patients: a single center study of incidence, clinical presentation and outcome. J Urol 2007;177:2300–5.
[21] Issler N, Dufek S, Kleta R, et al. Epidemiology of paediatric renal stone disease: a 22-year single centre experience in the UK. BMC Nephrol 2017;18:136.
[22] Tasian GE, Kabarrit AE, Kalmus A, et al. Kidney stone recurrence among children and adolescents. J Urol 2017;197(1):246–52.
[23] Sas DJ, Becton LJ, Tutman J, et al. Clinical, demographic, and laboratory characteristics of children with nephrolithiasis. Urolithiasis 2016;44:241–6.
[24] Kovacevic L, Wolfe-Christensen C, Edwards L, et al. From Hypercalciuria to hypocitraturia – a shifting trend in pediatric urolithiasis. J Urol 2012;188(4):1623–7.

[25] Alon US, Zimmerman H, Alon M. Evaluation and treatment of pediatric idiopathic urolithiasis - revisited. Pediatr Nephrol 2004;19:516–20.
[26] Meschi T, Maggiore U, Fiaccadori E, et al. The effect of fruits and vegetables on urinary stone risk factors. Kidney Int 2004;66:2402–10.
[27] Stapleton FB. Idiopathic hypercalciuria: association with isolated hematuria and risk for urolithiasis in children. Kidney Int 1990;37:807–11.
[28] Chu DI, Tasian GE, Copelovitch L. Pediatric kidney stones – avoidance and treatment. Curr Treat Option Pediatr 2016;2(2):104–11.
[29] Meschi T, Nouvenne A, Borghi L. Lifestyle recommendations to reduce the risk of kidney stones. Urol Clin North Am 2011;38:313–20.
[30] Curhan GC, Willett WC, Rimm EB, et al. A prospective study of dietary calcium and other nutrients and the risk of symptomatic kidney stones. N Engl J Med 1993;328:833–8.
[31] Tasian GE, Copelovitch L. Evaluation and medical management of kidney stones in children. J Urol 2014;192:1329–36.
[32] Borghi L, Schianchi T, Meschi T, et al. Comparison of two diets for the prevention of recurrent stones in idiopathic hypercalciuria. N Engl J Med 2002;346:77–84.
[33] Perminger GM, Sakhaee K, Skurla C, et al. Prevention of recurrent calcium stone formation with potassium citrate therapy in patients with distal renal tubular acidosis. J Urol 1985;134:20–3.
[34] Odvina CV. Comparative value of orange juice versus lemonade in reducing stone-forming risk. Clin J Am Soc Nephrol 2006;1:1269–74.
[35] Alon US. Medical treatment of pediatric urolithiasis. Pediatr Nephrol 2009;24(11):2129–35.
[36] Osorio AV, Alon US. The relationship between urinary calcium, sodium, and potassium excretion and the role of potassium in treating idiopathic hypercalciuria. Pediatrics 1997;100:675–81.
[37] Williams HE, Wandzilak TR. Oxalate synthesis, transport and the hyperoxaluric syndromes. J Urol 1989;141:742–9.
[38] Hoppe B, Beck BB, Milliner DS. The primary hyperoxalurias. Kidney Int 2009;75:1264–71.
[39] Neuhaus TJ, Belzer T, Blau N, et al. Urinary oxalate excretion in urolithiasis and nephrocalcinosis. Arch Dis Child 2000;82:322–6.
[40] Milliner DS, Eickholt JT, Bergstralh EJ, et al. Results of long-term treatment with orthophosphate and pyridoxine in patients with primary hyperoxaluria. N Engl J Med 1994;331:1553–8.
[41] Saravakos P, Kokkinou V, Giannatos E. Cystinuria: Current diagnosis and management. Urol 2014;83(4):693–9.
[42] Knoll T, Zöllner A, Wendt-Nordahl G, et al. Cystinuria in childhood and adolescence: recommendations for diagnosis, treatment, and follow-up. Pediatr Nephrol 2005;20:19–24.
[43] Kielb S, Koo HP, Bloom DA, et al. Nephrolithiasis associated with the ketogenic diet. J Urol 2000;164:464.
[44] Routh JC, Graham DA, Nelson CP. Trends in imaging and surgical management of pediatric urolithiasis at American pediatric hospitals. J Urol 2010;184(4):816–22.
[45] Salerno A, Nappo SG, Matarazzo E, et al. Treatment of pediatric renal stones in a western country: a changing pattern. J Pediatr Surg 2013;48(4):835–9.
[46] Long CJ, Srinivasan AK. Percutaneous nephrolithotomy and ureteroscopy in children: evolutions. Urol Clin North Am 2015;42(1):1–17.
[47] Assimos D, Krambeck A, Miller N, et al. Surgical Management of Stones: American Urologic Association/Endourological Society Guideline. 2016. Available at: https://www.auanet.org/guidelines/kidney-stones-surgical-management-guideline#x3164. Accessed November 16, 2019.
[48] Velazquez N, Zapata D, Wang HS. Medical expulsive therapy for pediatric urolithiasis: systematic review and meta-analysis. J Ped Urol 2015;11:321–7.

Advances in Pediatrics 67 (2020) 113–121
ADVANCES IN PEDIATRICS

Ovarian Masses and Torsion
New Approaches for Ovarian Salvage

Amy E. Lawrence, MD, Peter C. Minneci, MD, MHSc,
Katherine J. Deans, MD, MHSc*

Department of Pediatric Surgery, Center for Surgical Outcomes Research, Nationwide Children's Hospital, 700 Children's Drive, Columbus, OH 43205, USA

Keywords

• Ovary • Neoplasm • Torsion • Ovary-sparing surgery

Key points

- Work-up of ovarian neoplasms should include history, physical examination, imaging, and laboratory testing for tumor markers. These factors should all be included in evaluation of the patient for preoperative risk stratification to assist with deciding between ovary-sparing surgery and oophorectomy.
- Efforts to increase rates of ovary-sparing surgery for patients with low risk of malignancy include comprehensive evaluation of the patient and interdisciplinary collaboration if possible. Rates of ovary-sparing surgery for benign lesions are increasing.
- Ovarian torsion can be managed with detorsion alone because ovarian function is usually preserved after detorsion. The presence of a mass should not prompt oophorectomy because there is not an increased risk of malignancy. Compete work-up of a mass can be performed after detorsion.

INTRODUCTION

Ovarian lesions can be categorized into simple cysts and neoplasms. Simple cysts include diagnoses such as follicular and corpus luteal cysts, both of which may become hemorrhagic cysts. Although these lesions may rupture and cause significant pain, they are caused by normal physiologic function and are often referred to as functional or physiologic cysts [1,2]. In contrast, ovarian neoplasms refer to the abnormal growth of tissue and may arise from epithelial, germ cell, or sex cord/stromal tissues. These neoplasms may be benign or malignant.

*Corresponding author. *E-mail address:* Katherine.Deans@nationwidechildrens.org

https://doi.org/10.1016/j.yapd.2020.03.010

In addition to findings of cystic or neoplastic growth on the ovary, patients of all ages may experience ovarian torsion. When the ovary twists around its blood supply, it becomes ischemic, and emergent operative intervention is required to perform detorsion and salvage the ovary. An ovarian cyst or neoplasm may be identified in a patient with torsion and an operative decision for how to address the cyst or mass is needed.

Although ovarian neoplasms and torsion are rare occurrences in the pediatric population, recent research has provided new insights into the nature of these disease processes and helped shift practice patterns for surgeons. This article focuses on the diagnosis and management of both ovarian neoplasms and ovarian torsion.

RISK STRATIFICATION OF PEDIATRIC OVARIAN NEOPLASMS

The exact epidemiology of ovarian neoplasms among the pediatric population is unknown but is often estimated at around 2.2 per 100,000 patients [3]. Unlike adult patients, the risk of malignancy among pediatric patients presenting with an ovarian neoplasm is low. Studies have shown that malignancy is found in approximately 8% to 27% of ovarian masses among the pediatric population [3,4]. Mature teratomas and serous cystadenomas are the most common benign ovarian masses, and germ cell tumors are the most common malignant lesions [4,5]. However, differentiating between benign versus malignant tumors preoperatively remains a challenge. Evaluation of a patient with an ovarian neoplasm should include a thorough history and physical examination, laboratory testing, and imaging. Several recent studies have sought to identify various patient characteristics associated with increased risk of malignancy in order to assist with operative decision making [4,6–9].

Patient characteristics, symptoms, and physical examination

Patients with an ovarian mass often present with vague symptoms. Abdominal pain is a common chief complaint among patients with ovarian masses, but various studies have shown that it does not assist in differentiating between benign versus malignant masses [4,6,7,9]. Several studies have shown that abdominal bloating or findings of an abdominal mass were associated with an increased risk of malignancy, so the presence of either of these findings on physical examination in the setting of an ovarian mass warrants further evaluation [4,6,10,11]. Virilism or precocious puberty is another physical examination finding found to be associated with malignancy in a small number of studies [6,7]. Sex cord stromal tumors can secrete androgens, estrogens, or corticosteroids [12]. Therefore, a combination of an ovarian mass and symptoms of a hyperandrogenic or hyperestrogenic state should raise concern for possible sex cord stromal malignancy. In addition, although some studies have shown that ovarian masses in younger patients are more likely to be malignant, others have not shown any difference in rates of malignancy by age [3,4,6–10,13]. One limitation with regard to findings related to age is that many studies have different age criteria, and thus results should be interpreted within the parameters of each study. Notably, the physiology and natural course of ovarian masses identified in neonates is distinctly different from those identified in pediatric and adolescent patients, and is outside of the scope of this article [14]. Overall, there seems to be an increased risk of malignancy with younger age [10].

Imaging

Imaging of ovarian neoplasms is an important part of the preoperative workup. Most ovarian imaging is performed via either abdominal or transvaginal ultrasonography in sexually active patients, but computed tomography or MRI may be necessary if there is concern for malignancy. A variety of characteristics on imaging have been identified as concerning for malignancy and should help guide surgeons with regard to operative decision making.

Size has been shown to be an important factor in predicting malignancy, with larger neoplasms associated with higher risks of malignancy in multiple studies. The exact cutoff of when a mass is large enough to be concerning for malignancy varies slightly throughout the literature. One retrospective study by Rogers and colleagues [8] found that using a size cutoff of 8 cm for neoplasms resulted in a positive predictive value (PPV) of 37.1% and a negative predictive value (NPV) of 100%. A study by Papic and colleagues [9] found that tumors larger than or equal to 10 cm were associated with a 9.6 times greater likelihood of malignancy (univariate odds ratio [OR]; 95% confidence interval [CI], 2.12, 43.42). Another study showed that each 1-cm increase in lesion size was associated with a 12% increased odds of malignancy ($P<.001$) [15]. For tumor volume, a study by Abbas and colleagues [16] showed that volume may also play a role in predicting malignancy. Ovarian lesions with volumes of less than 184 cm^3 indicated benign disease with 100% sensitivity. Other imaging characteristics that have been found to be associated with increased odds of malignancy include solid components and the presence of lymphadenopathy [6,10]. A study by Stanković and colleagues [17] assessed the use of the Ueland morphology index and the presence of an ovarian crescent sign to predict malignancy. The Ueland morphology index uses components of tumor volume and wall structure to grade the likelihood of a mass being malignant [18]. The crescent sign is a radiologic finding indicating the presence of a ring of normal ovarian tissue [19]. Stanković and colleagues [17] found that a Ueland index of 7 or more and the absence of a crescent sign was highly predictive of malignancy, with a sensitivity of 93%, specificity of 97%, PPV of 85.7%, and an NPV of 98.9%.

There is no single finding that indicates malignancy, but imaging showing any of the previously mentioned radiologic features should be considered in conjunction with results of laboratory testing for ovarian tumor markers and the patient's initial presentation.

Laboratory testing

In addition to history, physical examination, and imaging, any patient who presents with an ovarian neoplasm should undergo laboratory testing for tumor markers. Studies have shown that an increased cancer antigen (CA) 125 level is associated with the presence of an epithelial ovarian malignancy [3,4,6,7,15]. However, unlike adults, most ovarian malignancies in children are not of epithelial origin, so additional laboratory testing is recommended. Beta human chorionic gonadotropin (beta-hCG) and alpha fetoprotein (AFP) are tumor markers commonly associated with germ cell tumors and the presence of malignancy [3,4,6,9,15]. Lactate dehydrogenase (LDH) is a common laboratory test for multiple inflammatory and malignant conditions and can also be used to detect ovarian malignancy [9,15]. An increased LDH level in the presence of an ovarian mass has a sensitivity of 95% for identification of malignancy but a specificity of only 13% [15]. More uncommonly tested tumor markers such as inhibin A and inhibin B have been found to have high specificity for malignancy (97% and 92%, respectively) [15]. Full results of sensitivity, specificity, PPV, and NPV for common tumor markers can be found in Table 1.

Importantly, none of these tumor markers alone offers high diagnostic accuracy. Given the variety of cell lines that give rise to ovarian malignancies in children, it is important to obtain tumor markers that represent different disorders. Papic and colleagues [9] found that increased levels of AFP, beta-hCG, and/or LDH resulted in a 225-fold increase in the odds of malignancy (95% CI, 34.65, >999). Given the high specificities of inhibin A and inhibin B, the authors recommend all patients with an ovarian neoplasm should undergo testing with a full panel of tumor markers, at a minimum including CA 125, AFP, beta-hCG, LDH, inhibin A, and inhibin B. Additional tumor marker testing may be appropriate and should be considered on a case-by-case basis.

Operative management

Results of laboratory testing, imaging, history, and physical examination should all be considered when determining whether to proceed with ovary-sparing

Table 1
Sensitivity, specificity, positive predictive value, and negative predictive values for increased tumor marker levels for any type of malignancy

Tumor marker	Sensitivity, % (95% CI)	Specificity, % (95% CI)	PPV, % (95% CI)	NPV, % (95% CI)
AFP	42% (31%–54%)	98% (97%–99%)	86% (75%–97%)	88% (84%–91%)
LDH	95% (89%–100%)	13% (6%–19%)	32% (24%–40%)	92% (81%–100%)
CEA	5% (0%–13%)	100% (100%–100%)	100% (100%–100%)	78% (70%–86%)
CA 125	59% (45%–72%)	81% (76%–87%)	49% (27%–62%)	87% (81%–92%)
CA 19-9	25% (0%–55%)	73% (60%–86%)	14% (0%–33%)	84% (73%–96%)
Beta-hCG	44% (32%–57%)	76% (71%–81%)	32% (22%–42%)	85% (80%–89%)
Inhibin A	32% (15%–49%)	97% (93%–100%)	82% (59%–100%)	80% (71%–88%)
Inhibin B	37% (19%–55%)	92% (86%–99%)	67% (43%–91%)	79% (70%–88%)

Abbreviation: CEA, carcinoembryonic antigen.

From Lawrence AE, Fallat ME, Hewitt G, et al. Understanding the Value of Tumor Markers in Pediatric Ovarian Neoplasms. *Journal of Pediatric Surgery*. 2019; with permission.

surgery (OSS) versus oophorectomy. Concern for malignancy warrants removal of the affected ovary and staging procedures according to the Children's Oncology Group guidelines [20]. However, patients with benign ovarian neoplasms experience a high rate of oophorectomies as well. Studies have shown that factors associated with increased rates of oophorectomy for benign disease include whether the patient was operated on by a pediatric surgeon or adult gynecologist (compared with a pediatric and adolescent gynecologist [PAG]), was younger, was admitted through the emergency department, had solid components on imaging, had a larger mass, or whether the mass was involved in a torsed ovary [10,21,22].

Several recent studies have proposed algorithms that incorporate various factors in order to preoperatively risk stratify patients for malignancy and thereby decrease rates of unnecessary oophorectomy while continuing to accurately identify malignancies [5,7,9,17,23]. A small number of these studies were completed prospectively, but, overall, data are limited. One study used quality improvement methodology to increase an institution's OSS rate from 28.8% to 96% without missing any ovarian malignancies [23]. A previous study has shown that the presence of an operating PAG at a hospital is associated with a significant increase in the rate of OSS for benign lesions [22]. Another study used a decision tree system to promote ovarian preservation. The system categorized treatment based on patient symptoms, menarchal status, CA 125 levels, and concern for malignancy based on imaging characteristics [7]. The first arm of their decision tree encouraged expectant management of patients who were asymptomatic and imaging consistent with a simple cyst. If the mass had concerning features on imaging and no crescent sign, it was treated as malignant. Their algorithm had a sensitivity of 93% and a specificity of 97% for predicting malignancy. The American Pediatric Surgical Association Outcomes and Evidence-based Practice Committee has also created an algorithm for the management of ovarian masses that advocates intraoperative frozen section in the setting of a mass with solid components and greater than or equal to 8 cm in size, greater than 185 cm^3 volume, Ueland index greater than or equal to 7, absent crescent sign, or any positive tumor markers from the panel of AFP, beta-hCG, LDH, CA 125, estradiol, and testosterone [5]. Although not prospectively evaluated, this algorithm proposes that definitive operative decisions should be made only after frozen section. This practice of using frozen section for decision making has only been reported on in 1 study focusing on pediatric patients, and this showed a congruency of frozen and final pathologic diagnosis of 55.1% for borderline or low-malignancy potential tumors [24].

Although there is no universal guideline for the preoperative evaluation of pediatric patients with ovarian masses, it is clear that operative decision making should be based on a review of the patient's history, physical examination, laboratory testing for tumor markers, and imaging findings. Which individual components and how much importance is given to each finding should be weighed on a case-by-case basis, and collaboration with various specialties has been shown to improve outcomes by avoiding unnecessary oophorectomies. An algorithm that uses imaging and laboratory results with evaluation of complex masses with concerning features by a multidisciplinary team consisting of a pediatric surgeon, a PAG, and a radiologist has been developed and is undergoing prospective multi-institutional evaluation (Fig. 1) [23].

OVARIAN TORSION

Ovarian torsion occurs when the ovary twists around its ligaments in the pelvis, cutting off blood supply to the organ. This acute event requires operative intervention to detorse the ovary, return it to its normal anatomic position, and restore its blood flow. However, this is a rare event in pediatric patients, with an estimated incidence of 4.9 in 100,000 patients [25]. One of the greatest challenges in ovarian torsion is preoperative diagnosis. Acute, severe pain is a common chief complaint [26]. A retrospective study by Melcer and colleagues [27] found that patients with torsion were more likely to present with nausea and vomiting and have signs of peritoneal irritation on physical examination

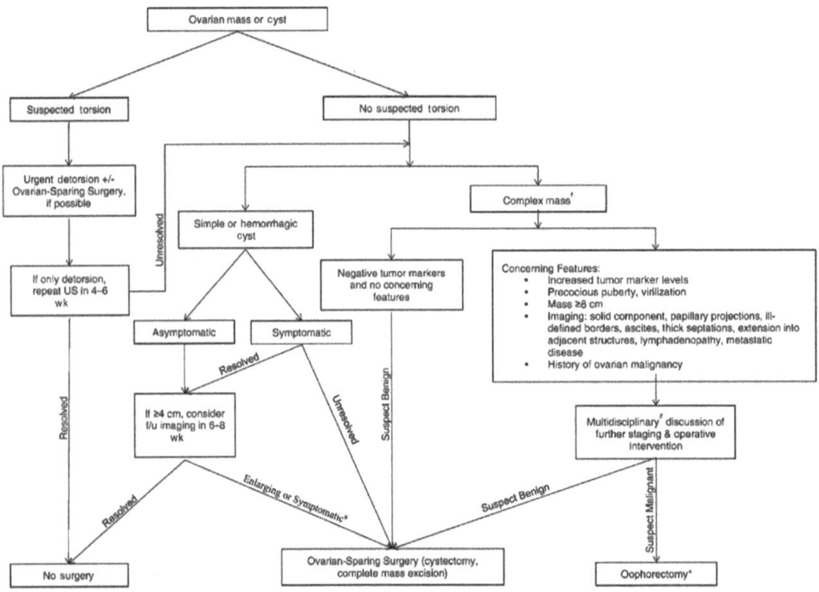

Fig. 1. Algorithm for the management of ovarian lesions. f/u, follow-up; US, ultrasonography. † Obtain tumor markers, including lactate dehydrogenase (LDH), alpha fetoprotein (AFP), beta human chorionic gonadotropin (β-HCG), inhibin A, cancer antigen 19-9 (CA19-9) and carcinoembryonic antigen (CEA), when applicable; # Pediatric Surgery, Pediatric and Adolescent Gynecology, Oncology Radiology, and Pathology; * Consider: Peritoneal washings; Inspection/biopsy of peritoneum, omentum, contralateral ovary, and retroperitoneal & pelvic lymph nodes; Salpingo-oophorectomy if unable to obtain negative margins with oophorectomy alone. (*From* Aldrink JH, Gonzalez DO, Sales SP, Deans KJ, Besner GE, Hewitt GD. Using quality improvement methodology to improve ovarian salvage for benign ovarian masses. *Journal of Pediatric Surgery.* 2018;53(1):67-72; with permission.)

than patients who were operated on for suspected torsion but found to have other disorders on diagnostic laparoscopy. When torsion is suspected, ultrasonography is often performed. However, definitive diagnosis of torsion via ultrasonography is difficult. A study by Peña and colleagues [28] in adult patients with torsion found that normal Doppler flow was detected in 60% of patients later confirmed to have torsion in the operating room, showing that ultrasonography is not able to accurately diagnose more than half of patients who present with torsion. Melcer and colleagues [27] found that patients with torsion were more likely to have enlargement of the ovary with signs of edema and free pelvic fluid.

Given the lack of definitive diagnosis via ultrasonography, clinical concern for torsion is an indication for diagnostic laparoscopy. Surgical practices vary once torsion is identified in the operating room. A Pediatric Health Information System study by Campbell and colleagues [29] identified that pediatric surgeons were significantly more likely to perform an oophorectomy for torsion compared with gynecologists (38% vs 27%; $P < .01$). However, a systematic review by Spinelli and colleagues [30] showed that ovarian preservation after torsion increased from 28% to 45% from 2000 to 2010, and recent studies report rates as high as 96% [31]. Oophoropexy is sometimes performed, but there is a lack of evidence to show that it reliably prevents recurrence [32]. Therefore, detorsion alone is recommended. Multiple studies have shown that, despite appearances of necrosis, most patients who undergo detorsion with ovarian preservation are found to have follicular development on postoperative imaging [33–36]. It is recommended that patients follow up with ultrasonography 4 to 6 weeks after detorsion in order to verify normalization of blood flow and volume of the ovary [35].

A subset of patients who present with torsion are found to have an associated ovarian lesion. These patients experience higher rates of oophorectomy than patients who present with torsion alone (OR, 2.16; 95% CI, 1.12–4.18) [10]. A study by Oltmann and colleagues [37] of rates of malignancy in patients who present with torsion found a rate of 1.8% compared with 10% of patients who presented with an ovarian mass without torsion. A multi-institutional study of more than 800 girls with ovarian neoplasms also did not identify torsion as a risk factor for malignancy [10]. These studies indicate that torsion should not increase suspicion for malignancy. If a mass is identified in the setting of torsion and cannot be safely removed from the ovary, detorsion alone with follow-up imaging 4 to 6 weeks postoperatively is recommended to further assess the characteristics of the mass and identify any concerning features for malignancy [32,33,35]. An approach of elective cystectomy once ischemia and edema are resolved following detorsion alone is an effective strategy.

SUMMARY

Although pediatric ovarian neoplasms and torsion are rare, recent research has provided significant information to help guide the evaluation and management of patients who present with these disorders. Preoperative risk stratification is possible with accuracy dependent on a comprehensive evaluation including a thorough history and physical examination, laboratory testing, and imaging. For most girls with an ovarian mass, ovarian preservation with OSS can be safely performed. In girls presenting with torsion, ovarian detorsion without oophorectomy is recommended regardless of the appearance of necrosis. In addition, in girls presenting with torsion and an ovarian mass, detorsion with either OSS (if the mass has a low likelihood of malignancy) or deferred resection of the mass until work-up is complete is recommended.

Disclosure

The authors have nothing to disclose.

References

[1] Liu JH, Zanotti KM. Management of the adnexal mass. Obstet Gynecol 2011;117(6): 1413–28.
[2] American College of Obstetricians and Gynecologists. ACOG Practice Bulletin. Management of adnexal masses. Obstet Gynecol 2007;110(1):201.
[3] Taskinen S, Fagerholm R, Lohi J, et al. Pediatric ovarian neoplastic tumors: incidence, age at presentation, tumor markers and outcome. Acta Obstet Gynecol Scand 2015;94(4): 425–9.
[4] Madenci AL, Levine B-S, Laufer MR, et al. Preoperative risk stratification of children with ovarian tumors. J Pediatr Surg 2016;51(9):1507–12.
[5] Renaud EJ, Sømme S, Islam S, et al. Ovarian masses in the child and adolescent: An American Pediatric Surgical Association Outcomes and Evidence-Based Practice Committee systematic review. J Pediatr Surg 2019;54(3):369–77.
[6] Oltmann SC, Garcia N, Barber R, et al. Can we preoperatively risk stratify ovarian masses for malignancy? J Pediatr Surg 2010;45(1):130–4.
[7] Depoers C, Martin F-A, Timoh KN, et al. A preoperative scoring system for adnexal mass in children and adolescents to preserve their future fertility. J Pediatr Adolesc Gynecol 2019;32(1):57–63.
[8] Rogers EM, Cubides GC, Lacy J, et al. Preoperative risk stratification of adnexal masses: can we predict the optimal surgical management? J Pediatr Adolesc Gynecol 2014;27(3): 125–8.
[9] Papic JC, Finnell SME, Slaven JE, et al. Predictors of ovarian malignancy in children: overcoming clinical barriers of ovarian preservation. J Pediatr Surg 2014;49(1):144–8.
[10] Lawrence AE, Gonzalez DO, Fallat ME, et al. Factors associated with management of pediatric ovarian neoplasms. Pediatrics 2019;144(1) [pii:e20182537].
[11] Hermans AJ, Kluivers KB, Wijnen MH, et al. Diagnosis and treatment of adnexal masses in children and adolescents. Obstet Gynecol 2015;125(3):611–5.
[12] Horta M, Cunha TM. Sex cord-stromal tumors of the ovary: a comprehensive review and update for radiologists. Diagn Interv Radiol 2015;21(4):277–86.
[13] Zhang M, Jiang W, Li G, et al. Ovarian masses in children and adolescents - an analysis of 521 clinical cases. J Pediatr Adolesc Gynecol 2014;27(3):e73–7.
[14] Dolgin SE. Ovarian masses in the newborn. Semin Pediatr Surg 2000;9(3):121–7.
[15] Lawrence AE, Fallat ME, Hewitt G, et al. Understanding the value of tumor markers in pediatric ovarian neoplasms. J Pediatr Surg 2020;55(1):122–5.
[16] Abbas PI, Elder SC, Mehollin-Ray AR, et al. Ovarian lesion volumes as a screening tool for malignancy in adolescent ovarian tumors. J Pediatr Surg 2015;50(11):1933–6.
[17] Stanković ZB, Sedlecky K, Savić D, et al. Ovarian preservation from tumors and torsions in girls: prospective diagnostic study. J Pediatr Adolesc Gynecol 2017;30(3):405–12.

[18] Ueland FR, DePriest PD, Pavlik EJ, et al. Preoperative differentiation of malignant from benign ovarian tumors: the efficacy of morphology indexing and Doppler flow sonography. Gynecol Oncol 2003;91(1):46–50.
[19] Stankovic ZB, Bjelica A, Djukic MK, et al. Value of ultrasonographic detection of normal ovarian tissue in the differential diagnosis of adnexal masses in pediatric patients. Ultrasound Obstet Gynecol 2010;36(1):88–92.
[20] Billmire D, Vinocur C, Rescorla F, et al. Outcome and staging evaluation in malignant germ cell tumors of the ovary in children and adolescents: an intergroup study. J Pediatr Surg 2004;39(3):424–9.
[21] Gonzalez DO, Cooper JN, Aldrink JH, et al. Variability in surgical management of benign ovarian neoplasms in children. J Pediatr Surg 2017;52(6):944–50.
[22] Trotman GE, Cheung H, Tefera EA, et al. Rate of oophorectomy for benign indications in a children's hospital: influence of a gynecologist. J Pediatr Adolesc Gynecol 2017;30(2): 234–8.
[23] Aldrink JH, Gonzalez DO, Sales SP, et al. Using quality improvement methodology to improve ovarian salvage for benign ovarian masses. J Pediatr Surg 2018;53(1):67–72.
[24] Song T, Choi CH, Lee Y-Y, et al. Pediatric borderline ovarian tumors: a retrospective analysis. J Pediatr Surg 2010;45(10):1955–60.
[25] Guthrie BD, Adler MD, Powell EC. Incidence and trends of pediatric ovarian torsion hospitalizations in the United States, 2000–2006. Pediatrics 2010;125(3):532.
[26] Rossi BV, Ference EH, Zurakowski D, et al. The clinical presentation and surgical management of adnexal torsion in the pediatric and adolescent population. J Pediatr Adolesc Gynecol 2012;25(2):109–13.
[27] Melcer Y, Maymon R, Pekar Zlotin M, et al. Clinical and sonographic predictors of adnexal torsion in pediatric and adolescent patients. J Pediatr Surg 2018;53(7):1396–8.
[28] Peña JE, Ufberg D, Cooney N, et al. Usefulness of Doppler sonography in the diagnosis of ovarian torsion. Fertil Steril 2000;73(5):1047–50.
[29] Campbell BT, Austin DM, Kahn O, et al. Current trends in the surgical treatment of pediatric ovarian torsion: we can do better. J Pediatr Surg 2015;50(8):1374–7.
[30] Spinelli C, Buti I, Pucci V, et al. Adnexal torsion in children and adolescents: new trends to conservative surgical approach–our experience and review of literature. Gynecol Endocrinol 2013;29(1):54–8.
[31] Adeyemi-Fowode O, Lin EG, Syed F, et al. Adnexal torsion in children and adolescents: a retrospective review of 245 cases at a single institution. J Pediatr Adolesc Gynecol 2019;32(1):64–9.
[32] Dasgupta R, Renaud E, Goldin AB, et al. Ovarian torsion in pediatric and adolescent patients: a systematic review. J Pediatr Surg 2018;53(7):1387–91.
[33] Walker SK, Lal DR, Boyd KP, et al. Management of pediatric ovarian torsion: evidence of follicular development after ovarian preservation. Surgery 2018;163(3):547–52.
[34] Geimanaite L, Trainavicius K. Ovarian torsion in children: Management and outcomes. J Pediatr Surg 2013;48(9):1946–53.
[35] Geimanaite L, Trainavicius K. Pediatric ovarian torsion: Follow- up after preservation of ovarian tissue. J Pediatr Surg 2019;54(7):1453–6.
[36] Aziz D, Davis V, Allen L, et al. Ovarian torsion in children: is oophorectomy necessary? J Pediatr Surg 2004;39(5):750–3.
[37] Oltmann SC, Fischer A, Barber R, et al. Pediatric ovarian malignancy presenting as ovarian torsion: incidence and relevance. J Pediatr Surg 2010;45(1):135–9.

Advances in Pediatrics 67 (2020) 123–129

ADVANCES IN PEDIATRICS

Approaches for Closing Gastroschisis

Charlene Dekonenko, MD[a], Jason D. Fraser, MD[a,b,*]

[a]Department of Surgery, Children's Mercy Kansas City, 2401 Gillham Road, Kansas City, MO 64108, USA; [b]University of Missouri Kansas City School of Medicine, 2411 Holmes Street, Kansas City, MO 64108, USA

Keywords

• Gastroschisis • Immediate closure • Delayed closure • Sutured closure • Sutureless closure • Silo

Key points

- The closure of gastroschisis can be performed immediately after birth or after gradual reduction of bowel over a number of days.
- The abdominal wall defect can be closed as a sutured fascial repair or as a sutureless repair using the umbilical cord as a biologic dressing.
- Owing to the low incidence and management variability, the optimal timing and closure method are still debated, and long-term outcomes are yet to be determined.

INTRODUCTION

Gastroschisis is a congenital defect of the anterior abdominal wall resulting in evisceration of the intestines with exposure to amniotic fluid. This condition is usually detected prenatally, and babies with gastroschisis can be born at or near term with expected survival of more than 90%. Morbidity is mostly determined by the severity of the bowel injury present at birth, and postnatal management goals include reduction of the bowel back into the abdominal cavity, closure of the abdominal wall defect, and initiation of enteral feeds. However, methods of obtaining abdominal wall closure vary and are still debated in the literature. Here we review and compare outcomes for the various approaches to closing gastroschisis.

*Corresponding author. School of Medicine, University of Missouri Kansas City, 2411 Holmes Street, Kansas City, MO 64108. *E-mail address:* jdfraser@cmh.edu

https://doi.org/10.1016/j.yapd.2020.03.005

IMMEDIATE VERSUS DELAYED CLOSURE

The timing for closure of gastroschisis varies, but reduction of the bowel and closure of the defect as soon as is feasible is optimal to prevent evaporative fluid loss, hypothermia, infection, and continued inflammation from exposure to the environment. However, returning the intestines to the abdominal cavity depends on multiple factors, including the state of the bowel (eg, edema, matting, ischemia) and the ability of the abdominal cavity to accommodate the viscera. Therefore, the timing of closure can be divided into 2 categories: immediate and delayed.

Immediate closure is performed at or shortly after birth, generally within the first 24 hours of life. Patients able to undergo immediate closure generally do not have significant matting or distension of intestinal loops and have enough abdominal domain to accommodate the bowel without creating excessive intra-abdominal pressure. Immediate closure can be performed in the operating room or at the bedside and has a reported success rate of 50% to 83% [1,2]. Potential advantages to immediate closure include prevention of further inflammation of the bowel from exposure and mechanical irritation, possible earlier initiation of feeds, a shorter hospital length of stay (LOS), and a decreased incidence of wound infection [3]. Potential disadvantages of immediate closure include an increase in days on the ventilator and requirement for nutritional support at discharge [3,4].

However, immediate closure is not always feasible. Patients with complex gastroschisis (atresia, necrosis, perforation) or with very thickened, distended bowel (matting), and little abdominal domain may require gradual reduction of the intestines and delayed closure of the defect. This process is accomplished using a silo technique where the eviscerated bowel is placed into a transparent, preformed silo and the spring-loaded or pliable ring at the base of the silo is placed into the abdomen through the defect. This procedure allows for gradual reduction of the intestines and enhancement of abdominal domain. Delayed closure with a premade silo obviates the need for the placement of sutures, thereby avoiding general anesthesia and allowing performance of the procedure at the bedside. Other advantages of delayed closure include a lower risk of abdominal compartment syndrome and a decrease in days on the ventilator [3,5]. The disadvantages of delayed closure include possible vascular compromise of the mesenteric vessels at the level of the defect owing to fascial compression from the silo, enlargement of the defect from the spring when duration of the silo is prolonged, and a longer hospital LOS [3,6,7].

SUTURED VERSUS SUTURELESS CLOSURE

The 2 common methods used to achieve abdominal wall closure are the sutured and sutureless methods. The traditional method is the sutured closure, whereas the more recent advancement is the sutureless closure technique. For a sutured closure, patients are taken to the operating room where a primary fascial repair is performed. The fascial defect, located to the right of the umbilicus, is closed with sutures either in an interrupted, running, or purse-string fashion. This skin is then closed around the umbilical stump so that it remains in a central position [3]. Sutured closure is sometimes preferred for patients with complex gastroschisis, because these patients may have atresia, perforation, or necrosis necessitating operative intervention, which incorporates abdominal wall closure into that operation.

In 2004, the sutureless abdominal wall closure method for gastroschisis was described. Sutureless closure allows reduction of the viscera at the bedside, at times without intubation and general anesthesia [3,8]. Once the bowel is reduced into the abdomen, the fascia at the site of the gastroschisis is left open, the umbilical cord is used to cover the defect, and an occlusive dressing is applied [9] (Fig. 1). The defect then contracts circumferentially leaving a normal-appearing umbilicus (Fig. 2). This method minimizes the increase in intra-abdominal pressure that occurs with fascial closure, decreasing, but not eliminating, the risk of abdominal compartment syndrome [3]. Proponents of the sutureless closure cite the avoidance of intubation and general anesthesia, the decreased ventilator days, the cost effectiveness of avoiding the operating room, and the enhanced cosmesis as reasons for transitioning clinical practice to primarily sutureless closure [7,10,11]. These findings were substantiated by a large retrospective multi-institutional study from

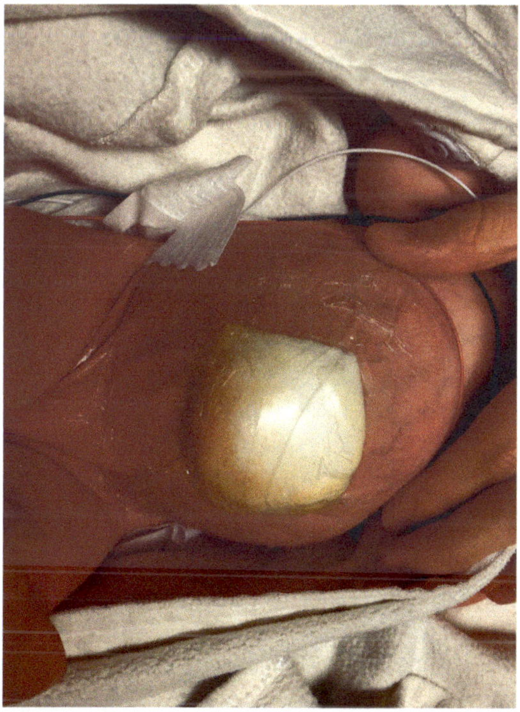

Fig. 1. Sutureless closure for gastroschisis.

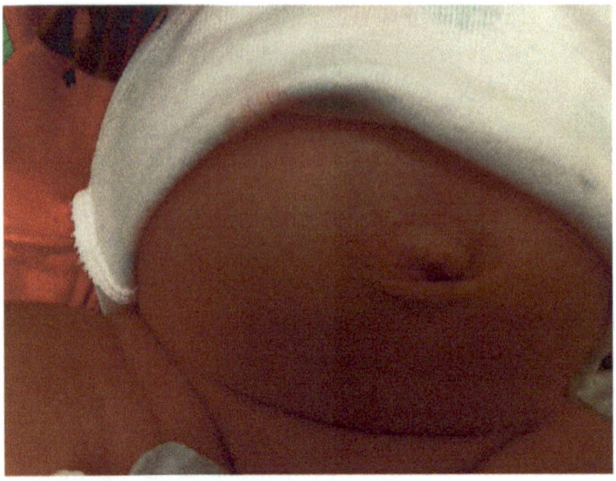

Fig. 2. Final result of sutureless closure for gastroschisis.

the Midwest Pediatric Surgery Consortium [12]. However, some investigators report a higher incidence of umbilical hernias with sutureless closure [10]. Whether these hernias need to be repaired, and at what age, is unclear because the long-term outcomes of this relatively new approach are yet to be determined. Such questions will be addressed in upcoming retrospective and prospective longitudinal studies through the Midwest Pediatric Surgery Consortium.

DISCUSSION

As with many congenital anomalies, the low incidence of gastroschisis limits the ability to obtain adequate data on outcomes at a single center. In contrast, variability in clinical practice among surgeons makes it difficult to interpret large, multicenter studies. Thus, the optimal timing and closure method are still debated and efforts to improve outcomes for these patients continue as the management of gastroschisis evolves.

Timing of gastroschisis closure

Generally, immediate closure is performed when achievable [5]. When immediate closure is not possible, delayed closure using a preformed silo is performed. With the advent of the preformed, spring-loaded silo, surgeons wondered whether it would be physiologically better to electively close the abdomen over a period of days. Thus, several studies have attempted to elucidate differences in outcomes between immediate closure versus initial silo placement and delayed closure. In a meta-analysis of studies in which randomization or temporal shifts in practice assigned patients to attempted primary closure or initial silo placement, silo placement was associated with a decrease in ventilator days, time to first feed, and rates of infection [13]. However, if studies are included where a silo was placed after failed primary closure, primary closure was associated with a shorter LOS, shorter parenteral nutrition duration, and fewer days on the ventilator, although the inherent selection bias toward worse clinical outcomes in those patients who failed primary closure and required a silo is evident [13].

In a study of 627 patients from the National Surgical Quality Improvement Program Pediatric database, delayed closure with silo placement was associated with an increased rate of surgical site infections and LOS, but a decreased number of ventilator days and less need for nutritional support at 30 days or at discharge [4]. In another even larger 4459 patient Pediatric Health Information System database study, delayed closure with silo placement was also associated with an increased LOS, and an increased duration of total parenteral nutrition requirement [14].

A multicenter, retrospective study comparing immediate versus delayed closure (<5 days) among 566 neonates across 8 institutions identified outcomes that were similar between the 2 approaches [15]. Multivariate analysis demonstrated that time to closure was an independent predictor of LOS, ventilator duration, time to full feeds, and total parenteral nutrition duration, which suggests that, whatever the approach, the sooner the defect can be closed, the better the outcome [15].

Sutured versus sutureless gastroschisis closure

Traditionally, the fascia at the site of the gastroschisis was closed with sutures at the time of reduction of the viscera. However, to do so requires bringing the muscle together, which produces increased abdominal wall tension and pressure. With the development of the sutureless approach, the fascia at the site of the gastroschisis is left open. Only the umbilical stump covers the defect, serving as the skin closure. Thus, sutureless closure of a gastroschisis is both cosmetically pleasing, and less invasive and, as a result, does not require general anesthesia nor the resources of an operating room. An early systematic review and meta-analysis comparing sutureless with sutured fascial closure revealed no differences in mortality, LOS, or duration of total parenteral nutrition. However, sutureless closure was associated with fewer wound infections and fewer days on the ventilator, although there was an increased risk of the development of an umbilical hernia [10]. A more recent meta-analysis found no difference in time to initiation of feeds, LOS, or mortality between the sutured and sutureless groups if they underwent immediate closure, but noted advantages to sutureless closure of gastroschisis after a silo was placed [16]. However, the authors acknowledged that the quality of the evidence reviewed was low for all outcomes.

The only existing prospective randomized trial comparing sutured with sutureless closure in 39 patients with gastroschisis revealed no difference in time to extubation, feeding complications, sepsis, or bowel operation, but an increase in LOS and a decrease in incidence of surgical site infections in the sutureless group [7]. Additional multi-institutional longitudinal studies are needed and such studies are underway to further guide optimal care of this complex and heterogenous patient population.

SUMMARY

The timing of closure for gastroschisis can be performed within hours of birth or delayed for several days using a preformed silo for gradual reduction of abdominal contents. However, the ability to perform immediate closure largely depends on the status of the bowel and the adequacy of abdominal domain. The necessity to delay closure in some patients with gastroschisis has contributed to the evolution of the preformed silo that allows bedside reduction without the need for an operation and general anesthesia. Naturally, studies have sought to compare outcomes in immediate versus delayed closure. The overarching consensus in the current literature suggests that outcomes in patients who undergo early closure, either immediate or within 5 days, are improved compared with those whose closure is delayed for longer periods of time. Evidence for the superiority of closure method, either sutured or sutureless, is less clear. Existing retrospective studies suggest fewer ventilator days, less anesthetic use, and fewer surgical site infections in patients managed with the sutureless approach. However, the only existing prospective randomized trial only detected a difference in wound infection rates favoring sutureless repair and LOS favoring the sutured approach. These conflicting data are likely due to heterogeneity in study populations, variability in clinical practice, and continual evolution in postnatal management of gastroschisis. With the rising incidence of gastroschisis, efforts should be focused on standardization of postnatal care to better study this unique population and improve outcomes.

Disclosure

No disclosures.

References

[1] Henrich K, Huemmer HP, Reingruber B, et al. Gastroschisis and omphalocele: treatments and long-term outcomes. Pediatr Surg Int 2008;24:167–73.
[2] Driver CP, Bruce J, Bianchi A, et al. The contemporary outcome of gastroschisis. J Pediatr Surg 2000;35:1719–23.
[3] Petrosyan M, Sandler AD. Closure methods in gastroschisis. Semin Pediatr Surg 2018;27: 304–8.
[4] Gurien LA, Dassinger MS, Burford JM, et al. Does timing of gastroschisis repair matter? A comparison using the ACS NSQIP pediatric database. J Pediatr Surg 2017;52:1751–4.
[5] Skarsgard ED. Management of gastroschisis. Curr Opin Pediatr 2016;28:363–9.
[6] Ryckman J, Aspirot A, Laberge JM, et al. Intestinal venous congestion as a complication of elective silo placement for gastroschisis. Semin Pediatr Surg 2009;18:109–12.
[7] Bruzoni M, Jaramillo JD, Dunlap JL, et al. Sutureless vs sutured gastroschisis closure: a prospective randomized controlled trial. J Am Coll Surg 2017;224:1091–6.
[8] Pet GE, Stark RA, Meehan JJ, et al. Outcomes of bedside sutureless umbilical closure without endotracheal intubation for gastroschisis repair in surgical infants. Am J Surg 2017;213: 958–62.
[9] Sandler A, Lawrence J, Meehan J, et al. A "plastic" sutureless abdominal wall closure in gastroschisis. J Pediatr Surg 2004;39:738–41.
[10] Youssef F, Gorgy A, Arbash G, et al. Flap versus fascial closure for gastroschisis: a systematic review and meta-analysis. J Pediatr Surg 2016;51:718–25.
[11] Grabski DF, Hu Y, Vavolizza RD, et al. Sutureless closure: a versatile treatment for the diverse presentations of gastroschisis. J Perinatol 2019;39:666–72.

[12] Fraser JD, Deans KJ, Fallat ME. Midwest Pediatric Surgery Consortium. Sutureless vs sutured abdominal wall closure for gastroschisis: Operative characteristics and early outcomes from the Midwest Pediatric Surgery Consortium. J Pediatr Surg 2020; https://doi.org/10.1016/j.jpedsurg.2020.02.017. [Epub ahead of print].
[13] Kunz SN, Tieder JS, Whitlock K, et al. Primary fascial closure versus staged closure with silo in patients with gastroschisis: a meta-analysis. J Pediatr Surg 2013;48:845–57.
[14] Gonzalez DO, Cooper JN, St. Peter SD, et al. Variability in outcomes after gastroschisis closure across U.S. children's hospitals. J Pediatr Surg 2018;53:513–20.
[15] Hawkins RB, Raymond SL, St. Peter SD, et al. Immediate versus silo closure for gastroschisis: results of a large multicenter study. J Pediatr Surg 2019 [pii:S0022-3468(19)30509-3].
[16] Miyake H, Seo S, O'Connell JS, et al. Safety and usefulness of plastic closure in infants with gastroschisis: a systematic review and meta-analysis. Pediatr Surg Int 2019;35:107–16.

Advances in Pediatrics 67 (2020) 131–143

ADVANCES IN PEDIATRICS

Inguinal and Other Hernias

Aimee G. Kim, MD[a], Marcus D. Jarboe, MD[a,b,*]

[a]Section of Pediatric Surgery, Department of Surgery, University of Michigan, Mott Children's Hospital, 1540 East Hospital Drive SPC 4217, Ann Arbor, MI 48109 - 4217, USA; [b]Division of Vascular and Interventional Radiology, Department of Radiology, University of Michigan, Mott Children's Hospital, 1540 East Hospital Drive SPC 4217, Ann Arbor, MI 48109 - 4217, USA

Keywords

• Inguinal hernia • Minimally invasive pediatric inguinal hernia repair
• Neonatal hernia • Umbilical hernia

Key points

- An indirect inguinal hernia is a common cause for evaluation, with a higher incidence in boys and premature/low birth weight infants.
- Benefits of early repair include avoiding the risk of incarceration/strangulation versus the benefits of delayed repair include minimizing the cardiopulmonary risks of anesthesia and decreasing the risk of recurrence.
- There is variability among pediatric surgeons with regards to exploring the contralateral side; the risk of developing a hernia with a patent processus vaginalis is low.
- No differences were found between laparoscopy and open repair of inguinal hernias with regards to postoperative complications, hospital length of stay, or time of recovery.
- Most pediatric umbilical hernias should close spontaneously. Symptomatic hernias should be repaired. Otherwise, repair can be delayed to 4 years of age.

INTRODUCTION

Hernias in the pediatric population, and especially in the neonate, are a common cause for evaluation by pediatricians and pediatric surgeons. In children, most abdominal wall hernias arise as a congenital defect of embryologic development. In this article, we review various pediatric hernia diagnoses with a

*Corresponding author. Mott Children's Hospital, 1540 East Hospital Drive SPC 4217, Ann Arbor, MI 48109 - 4217. *E-mail address:* marjarbo@med.umich.edu

https://doi.org/10.1016/j.yapd.2020.03.009
0065-3101/20/

focus on the inguinal hernia, current topics of controversy, and updates to surgical management in the era of minimally invasive techniques.

INDIRECT INGUINAL HERNIA

Embryology

The inguinal hernia in the neonate is the result of an arrest of normal embryologic development. Beginning around 12 weeks of gestation, a "finger" of peritoneum enters the inguinal canal and descends into the scrotum as the processus vaginalis in boys. This process is followed by descent of the testes between 28 and 36 weeks of gestation. The processus then closes and is obliterated by 36 to 40 weeks of gestation, although 40% of patent processus vaginalis may close within the first few months of life [1]. The left testis descends before the right, and the left processus closes before that of the right. A persistent patent processus vaginalis does not necessitate a hernia, although most congenital inguinal hernias are preceded by a patent processus. The contents of the space determine the diagnosis: omentum, bowel, or ovary define an inguinal hernia, whereas freely communicating peritoneal fluid defines a communicating hydrocele [2,3].

Epidemiology

The cumulative incidence of inguinal hernias in children aged 0 to 15 years is a reported 7% in males and 1% in females in a large population-based study [4]. The incidence in males peaks in infancy (<1 year of age), whereas in females, the incidence peaks at 5 years of age. The ratio of unilateral to bilateral hernias is 5:1, and females have bilateral hernias almost twice as often as males (25% vs 13%).

Preterm infants

Preterm infants comprise an important subset in the discussion of pediatric inguinal hernias and their management. Not only are preterm infants more likely to be diagnosed with inguinal hernias (16%–31% diagnosed among extremely low birth weight [<1000 g] and very low birth weight [<1500 g] neonates) [5,6], they have a higher rate of incarceration compared with their term counterparts (11% vs 7%) [7], and higher complication rates related to surgery (28% vs 12%) [8].

The risk of incarceration and associated complications weighed against the operative and perioperative risks associated with intervention in preterm low birth weight neonates is an ongoing point of discussion with regards to timing of operation (before discharge from the neonatal intensive care unit [NICU] vs electively after discharge) (Table 1). A survey of pediatric surgeons in the Section on Surgery of the American Academy of Pediatrics in 2003 reported that 63% would repair a reducible inguinal hernia in a former 29-week 1000-g patient before discharge from the NICU [9]. In the same survey, 53% would repair a reducible hernia in a preterm infant already discharged from the NICU "when convenient, regardless of age." Approximately one-half (49%) would not delay repair for a coexisting condition, whereas 37% would delay

Table 1
Benefits to inguinal hernia surgery in the preterm neonate before versus after discharge from the NICU

Before NICU discharge	After NICU discharge
Avoids risk of incarceration, strangulation, testicular atrophy	Minimizes cardiopulmonary risks of anesthesia in younger gestational age
Decreases risk of surgical complications	Decreases the risk of recurrence
Decreased adhesions between hernia sac and spermatic cord	There is potential for spontaneous resolution
Combines with other surgical procedures	Decreases technical challenges of operating on smaller neonate
Avoids a readmission for surgery	

for concurrent bronchopulmonary dysplasia with oxygen requirement, 32% for apneic/bradycardic episodes on home monitors, and 15% for well-managed cardiac disease. These statistics reveal the lack of clear evidence and consensus on the optimal timing for inguinal hernia repair in the former preterm neonate, or even the criteria that should determine optimal timing. To address this question, there is currently a randomized controlled clinical trial underway specifically comparing the safety of inguinal hernia repair in the preterm neonate before NICU discharge versus delay to 55 to 60 weeks postmenstrual age (ClinicalTrials.gov Identifier: NCT01678638).

The arguments favoring early repair before discharge from the NICU include avoiding the risk of incarceration, strangulation, and the associated risk of gonadal infarction, all complications more prevalent in the preterm neonate [10,11]. The increased risk of surgical complications with early repair may be related to the fragility of the hernia sac and the spermatic cord [12]. An analysis of a large administrative dataset revealed that the time interval from birth to repair did not affect the risk of incarceration in premature infants, but a delay to more than 40 weeks postconceptual age doubled the risk of incarceration [13].

A recent systematic review and meta-analysis of 6 studies investigating repair before and after discharge from the NICU found no significant difference in incarceration rates or in surgical complication rates between the 2 groups [14]. There was, however, a statistically significant difference for inguinal hernia recurrence and postoperative respiratory difficulties favoring delayed repair.

Additional arguments for delayed repair, in elective fashion after discharge from the NICU, include minimizing the cardiopulmonary risks of anesthesia, more favorable technical conditions in a larger infant, and the chance of spontaneous resolution. Postoperative apnea is strongly and inversely related to both gestational age and postconceptional age [15]. Delaying surgery and using spinal or regional anesthesia may decrease the risks of clinically significant apneic events postoperatively in former preterm infants [16,17]. In 2 different institutional studies, preterm infants who underwent inguinal hernia repair before discharge had longer postoperative ventilator dependence and postoperative hospital stays compared with their counterparts who underwent delayed elective repair [18,19]. Results from a large pediatric database reported more critical care interventions, higher readmission rates, and higher reoperation rates at 1 year in the early repair group [11]. Spontaneous resolution or disappearance of an inguinal hernia is a very rare occurrence described in small numbers in a large series (1%) [20].

Diagnosis

A bulge in the inguinal–scrotal region in the pediatric patient most commonly may be an inguinal hernia, a communicating hydrocele, or a noncommunicating hydrocele [21]. Features of the clinical history and physical examination should be consistent with the diagnosis. A history of a painless bulge that does not change in size with position, time of day, or increased intra-abdominal pressure favors a noncommunicating hydrocele. An inguinal hernia or communicating hydrocele more often presents with a history of variability in size and intermittent and spontaneous reduction or resolution, and is found to be more apparent with crying, standing, daytime, or increased intra-abdominal pressure. In the case of an incarcerated inguinal hernia, a bulge that was historically intermittent may present with an inability to be reduced, with associated irritability, tenderness, and/or signs of intestinal obstruction [3].

Physical examination should begin with identifying the bulge, if present, and determining the proximal and distal extent. If cord structures are palpable proximal to a distinct oblong-shaped bulge along the inguinal canal and bilateral testes are appropriately located in the scrotum, a hydrocele may be suspected [3]. Distinguishing a communicating hydrocele versus an inguinal hernia can sometimes be challenging, but palpation should differentiate between reduction of fluid versus intra-abdominal contents. In the diagnosis of an inguinal hernia, the classic "silk stocking" or "silk glove" sign refers to gently rolling the fingertips near the pubic tubercle and feeling the hernia sac slipping on itself like silk rubbing on silk alongside the normal cord structures [2].

The role of ultrasound examination is limited, and at times can be misleading, in the diagnosis of the neonatal or pediatric inguinal hernia; most diagnoses are able to be determined by a good history and physical examination. The application of ultrasound examination in the management of pediatric inguinal hernias gained traction in the 1990s when alternatives to preemptive surgical exploration of the contralateral side were being investigated. Ultrasound examination may be a useful adjunct, but only in unusual circumstances where the diagnosis remains unclear. Standardized criteria do not exist currently for ultrasound examination in the diagnosis of an inguinal hernia and the use of this modality is not considered a routine, cost-effective practice [22]. With regard to using ultrasound examination in the preoperative setting to predict a contralateral inguinal hernia, a recent review and meta-analysis suggested that although it may identify a contralateral patent processus vaginalis with accuracy, it may also overestimate contralateral hernia prevalence [23].

Surgical intervention

Repair of the reducible inguinal hernia occurs in elective fashion shortly after diagnosis in the term neonate. Diagnosis or suspicion of a communicating hydrocele in the absence of a definite hernia is treated most often like an inguinal hernia, with 46% of surveyed pediatric surgeons choosing to repair electively [9]. The natural history of a noncommunicating hydrocele has not been studied beyond 2 years of age. However, the majority are likely to spontaneously resolve, and, therefore, elective repair is often delayed to 1 to 2 years of age. There is no evidence for risk of testicular damage from delaying repair. The only indication for early repair is a concomitant diagnosis of an inguinal hernia [24,25].

The risk of incarceration for an inguinal hernia is reported to be 7% to 9% and is the main indication for operative intervention [7,26]. More than one-third of cases presenting with incarceration in 2 series were previously diagnosed and awaiting surgical repair. A large majority are able to be manually reduced (84%) with steady pressure and minimal sedation and/or analgesia [26]. Thus, bedside manual reduction should be attempted in cases in which there is no concern for bowel compromise, peritonitis, or hemodynamic instability. Potential complications related to incarceration range from 9% to 30% and include wound infection, gonadal infarction, hernia recurrence, and bowel resection [7,8,21,27]. Surgical repair is recommended to be performed during the same hospitalization in those who present with incarceration after successful manual reduction, with laparoscopic evaluation of the bowel to ensure viability only when there is clinical concern for bowel ischemia. Incarcerated inguinal hernias that are unable to be reduced should proceed emergently to operative reduction.

Surgical approaches

The traditional open repair of the pediatric indirect inguinal hernia with high ligation of the hernia sac is attributed to Potts and Czerny [2]. In the largest and longest series of patients with inguinal hernias operated on by a single surgeon using open technique, (6361 patients over 35 years), 1.2% experienced a recurrence, 1.2% had a wound infection, and 0.3% had testicular atrophy postoperatively.

Despite being one of the most common surgeries performed in children, there is no universally acknowledged standard technique for open repair of the pediatric inguinal hernia, and there is considerable variability among pediatric surgeons with regard to specific practices [28]. In a survey of 447 pediatric surgeons from 2002%, 81% could trace their hernia approach lineage to Drs Ladd and Gross, but many report practice that differs from the original description, likely attributed to evolving techniques and application of new knowledge as well as the experience and teaching of immediate surgical mentors [29,30].

With the advent of laparoscopy, numerous variations on the minimally invasive approach have been proposed and described. Ostlie and Ponsky (2014) [31] provide a good summary of various laparoscopic techniques, as well as their preferred modification. Generally, the laparoscopic approaches can be categorized by the method used to close the internal ring: intraperitoneal approaches (intracorporeal suturing) or extraperitoneal approaches (suture through the abdominal wall). The intraperitoneal techniques generally involve a laparoscopic approach wherein the hernia sac is either cauterized or circumferentially divided, with care to avoid injury to the vas deferens and the testicular vessels, followed by intracorporeal placement of a purse string suture to close the peritoneum and, thus, to obliterate the sac opening. The extraperitoneal techniques involves using various types of needles under laparoscopic guidance to percutaneously secure a suture circumferentially around the internal ring, thus, again, obliterating the sac opening.

Still, 83% of pediatric surgeons favor open repair [32]. There have been a number of studies that have compared open and laparoscopic approaches, with 1 recent literature analysis covering the last 20 years reporting no significant difference in (1) operative time for repair of a unilateral inguinal hernia or (2) recurrence rates [33]. Operative time for repair of a bilateral hernia was significantly less with laparoscopy, however, and rates of other complications such as wound infection, postoperative hydrocele formation, iatrogenic cryptorchidism, and testicular atrophy were significantly increased with open repair. Two recent meta-analyses of studies ranging from 2005 to 2018 corroborated some, but not all, of these results [34,35]. No differences were found between laparoscopy and open repair with regard to postoperative complications (recurrences, infection, hydrocele, testicular atrophy, hematoma, seroma, or pain), hospital length of stay, or time of recovery. Laparoscopy resulted in superior wound appearance and was also faster for repair of bilateral inguinal hernias. Comparing intraperitoneal and extraperitoneal laparoscopic approaches versus open repair for a unilateral inguinal hernia, the extraperitoneal approach was faster than open repair, but open repair was faster than the intraperitoneal approach.

The newest development to minimally invasive hernia repair is inguinal herniorrhaphy using ultrasound guidance [36]. In this novel approach, the inguinal hernia is first manually reduced under ultrasound imaging and a hollow needle is passed under ultrasound guidance through the skin, first lateral to the hernia, then under and around, and then out through the skin medial to the hernia (Fig. 1). A silk suture is passed through the needle and the needle is removed. The needle is then passed through the same skin insertion and exit sites, the only difference being the needle tract passes over and superficial to the hernia (as opposed to under). The same suture is passed through the needle from medial to lateral, and the needle is removed. The suture then has formed a loop circumferentially around the hernia defect (Fig. 2). The silk suture is then tied down, and a needle laparoscope is placed to confirm appropriate placement of the suture. Initial results in a series of 15 female patients

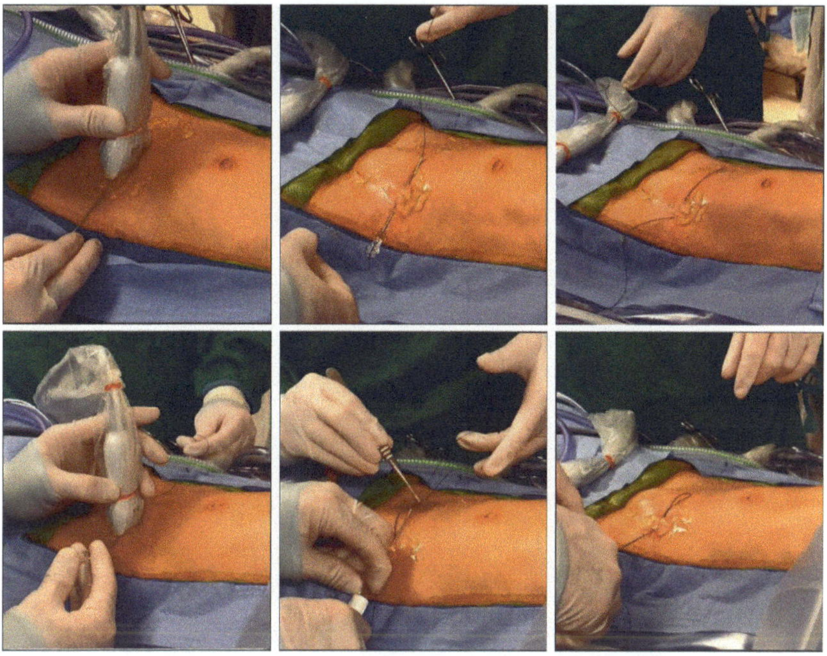

Fig. 1. Ultrasound-guided inguinal herniorrhaphy. First, the inguinal hernia is manually reduced and confirmed on ultrasound examination. A hollow needle is then passed under ultrasound guidance from lateral to medial, traversing deep to the hernia sac, avoiding the iliac and epigastric vessels, and exiting the skin medial to the hernia sac. A silk suture is passed through the needle and the needle is removed. The needle is used to pass through the same skin insertion and exit sites a second time, under ultrasound guidance, and this time traversing superficial to the hernia sac. The same suture is passed through the needle, forming a loop to encircle the hernia sac. In these pilot experiments, the suture was tied down and a needle laparoscope used to confirm obliteration of the hernia defect.

demonstrated the technique was safe and effective. Three cases were converted to laparoscopic repair secondary to sliding components seen on ultrasound imaging, and there were no recurrences in short-term follow-up. A larger study is needed with longer follow-up. However, in the future, this technique could be performed without laparoscopic confirmation and under sedation to avoid general anesthesia.

Contralateral exploration

In 1955, Rothenberg and Barnett recommended a "prophylactic" exploration of the contralateral groin [37], and scores of subsequent publications have reported on the incidence of a contralateral patent processus vaginalis and its implications on the risk of metachronous contralateral hernias. The natural history of a patent processus vaginalis is unclear. In a review of the literature over the last 2 decades, the incidence of contralateral processus vaginalis

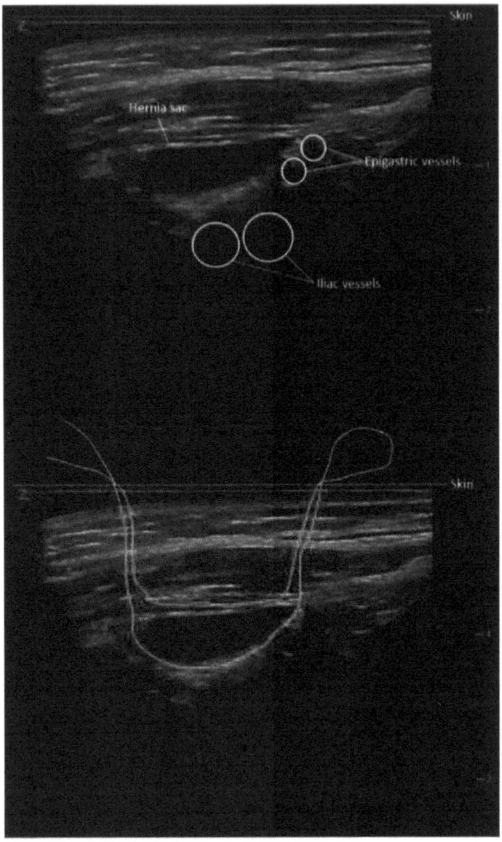

Fig. 2. (*Top*) Ultrasound image of an indirect hernia sac with associated vascular structures labeled (epigastric vessels laterally and iliac vessels deep to the sac). (*Bottom*) The blue line depicts the course of the suture that is tied down to ligate the sac and obliterate the defect.

patency ranged from 20% to 66% [33]. Incidence differs by gender and gestational age and, in a study of infants less than 6 months of age, the highest incidence of a contralateral patent processus vaginalis occurred in term and preterm female infants with a left-sided hernia [38].

A prospective analysis of 1548 infants and children undergoing nonhernia laparoscopy demonstrated that 20% had a patent processus vaginalis at a median of 5 years of age [39]. Six percent developed an inguinal hernia in follow-up compared with 0.5% in those without a patent processus vaginalis. Even so, this risk is low in light of the reported frequency of patent processus vaginalis, especially in infants. Currently, prophylactic repair is not recommended. The MidWest Pediatric Surgery Consortium is currently following those infants with patent processus vaginalis identified at the time of laparoscopic pyloromyotomy to ascertain the risk of clinically symptomatic inguinal hernia in the setting of patent processus vaginalis.

In a meta-analysis looking at the incidence of metachronous contralateral inguinal hernia after unilateral repair, 6% of children developed a contralateral hernia [40]. An initial left-sided hernia and a contralateral patent processus vaginalis were found to be risk factors. Complications from contralateral exploration are reported to range from 2% to 16% and include wound infection, hematoma, injury to spermatic cord structures (vas deferens, nerve, testicular atrophy, acquired undescended testes), injury to intraperitoneal structures (eg, intestine, ovary), and injury to epigastric or femoral vessels [21,41]. There is no consensus recommendation with regard to if or when to consider contralateral exploration, but fewer than one-half of pediatric surgeons (44% in males $\leq$2 years old, 47% in females of $\leq$4 years old) reported this as a routine practice in 2003 compared with 1993 (65% and 84%, respectively) [9]. Peritoneoscopy through the inguinal hernia sac during open repair as well as laparoscopy at the time of laparoscopic repair of an inguinal hernia are often used to assess for a patent processus vaginalis and repair performed when one is identified.

UMBILICAL HERNIA

All neonates have a defect at the umbilicus through which the umbilical vessels traverse. This defect closes spontaneously in the majority during the early days to weeks of infancy. An umbilical hernia is present in 15% to 23% of newborns, and the incidence is higher in premature and low birth weight infants compared with term infants [42]. In a recent systematic review, a large majority of umbilical hernias (>90%) close spontaneously without surgical intervention within the first couple of years of life [43]. Thus, it is unusual to repair an asymptomatic umbilical hernia in a patient less than 2 years of age. Among those not undergoing surgical repair, complications are rare in the United States, with incarceration rates ranging from 0.2% to 5.0%, but more likely to be in the 1% range. The data are conflicting with regard to the relationship between the size of the defect and complication rates. In a retrospective single-institution study of more than 5 decades of umbilical hernia management, the mean defect size for complicated cases necessitating emergent repair was significantly smaller compared with elective cases (1.0 cm emergent vs 1.5 cm elective). Recommendations for the timing of operative repair ranged from 2 years of age to 10 years of age or older in the systematic review, with some reports giving special consideration for early repair (eg, limited access to health care, size of the defect). The authors of the systematic review suggested a consensus target of more than 4 years of age for repair of the asymptomatic umbilical hernia because a majority of reports concluded that there was no increased risk of complications in patients less than 4 years of age and there may be associated risks to long-term neurodevelopment (the data are mixed) [44,45] and respiratory complications [46] with anesthetic exposure in younger patients.

Surgical repair of the pediatric umbilical hernia is usually performed open via a curvilinear infraumbilical incision. Various techniques for pediatric umbilical hernia repair have been described, but no studies have compared them. In a retrospective study of more than 50 years of pediatric umbilical hernia repairs in a single institution with mailed surveys for follow-up (response rate 66%), 2% reported a recurrence, 90% reported satisfaction with cosmesis, and 96% reported being pain free [47].

EPIGASTRIC HERNIA

Epigastric hernias or congenital ventral hernias are usually superior to the umbilicus and the result of failure of the linea alba to approximate in the midline during the final stages of abdominal wall development. They comprise 4% of all pediatric hernias and approximately one-half are symptomatic or enlarging [48]. Surgical repair is recommended in an elective fashion, usually performed via an open approach. An ultrasound-guided approach has also been described, performed similarly as for the inguinal hernia, with promising short-term results in a pilot series, but will require longer follow-up [49]. The defect is usually small (1–2 mm in diameter), and a palpable mass is usually composed of herniated preperitoneal fat. It is important to mark the site of the bulge while the patient is awake because identification of the defect may be difficult after induction of anesthesia [2].

RARE PEDIATRIC HERNIAS

Direct inguinal hernias and femoral hernias are a rare occurrence in the pediatric population with a reported incidence of 0.2% to 2.0% and 0.2% to 1.0%, respectively [50,51]. These hernias are difficult to diagnose clinically, and recently more are being identified with the advent of laparoscopy and laparoscopic repair of inguinal hernias. Both direct and femoral hernias have been found in the setting of recurrence after open inguinal hernia repair (which may have been misdiagnoses initially). Repair is recommended using a tissue-only approach, and have been performed using both open and laparoscopic techniques [2,52].

SUMMARY

Despite being a common diagnosis and procedure, there is still significant variability in practice patterns with regards to surgical management of pediatric hernias, especially in the former preterm infant with an inguinal hernia.

Disclosure

The authors have nothing to disclose.

References

[1] Rowe MI, Copelson LW, Clatworthy HW. The patent processus vaginalis and the inguinal hernia. J Pediatr Surg 1969;4(1):102–7.
[2] Brandt ML. Pediatric hernias. Surg Clin North Am 2008;88(1):27–43, vii-viii.
[3] Palmer LS. Hernias and hydroceles. Pediatr Rev 2013;34(10):457–64 [quiz: 464].
[4] Chang SJ, Chen JY, Hsu CK, et al. The incidence of inguinal hernia and associated risk factors of incarceration in pediatric inguinal hernia: a nation-wide longitudinal population-based study. Hernia 2016;20(4):559–63.

[5] Harper RG, Garcia A, Sia C. Inguinal hernia: a common problem of premature infants weighing 1,000 grams or less at birth. Pediatrics 1975;56(1):112–5.
[6] Rajput A, Gauderer MWL, Hack M. Inguinal hernias in very low birth weight infants: incidence and timing of repair. J Pediatr Surg 1992;27(10):1322–4.
[7] Olesen CS, Mortensen LQ, Oberg S, et al. Risk of incarceration in children with inguinal hernia: a systematic review. Hernia 2019;23(2):245–54.
[8] Baird R, Gholoum S, Laberge J-M, et al. Prematurity, not age at operation or incarceration, impacts complication rates of inguinal hernia repair. J Pediatr Surg 2011;46(5):908–11.
[9] Antonoff MB, Kreykes NS, Saltzman DA, et al. American Academy of Pediatrics Section on Surgery hernia survey revisited. J Pediatr Surg 2005;40(6):1009–14.
[10] Vaos G, Gardikis S, Kambouri K, et al. Optimal timing for repair of an inguinal hernia in premature infants. Pediatr Surg Int 2010;26(4):379–85.
[11] Sulkowski JP, Cooper JN, Duggan EM, et al. Does timing of neonatal inguinal hernia repair affect outcomes? J Pediatr Surg 2015;50(1):171–6.
[12] Uemura S, Woodward AA, Amerena R, et al. Early repair of inguinal hernia in premature babies. Pediatr Surg Int 1999;15(1):36–9.
[13] Lautz TB, Raval MV, Reynolds M. Does timing matter? a national perspective on the risk of incarceration in premature neonates with inguinal hernia. J Pediatr 2011;158(4):573–7.
[14] Masoudian P, Sullivan KJ, Mohamed H, et al. Optimal timing for inguinal hernia repair in premature infants: a systematic review and meta-analysis. J Pediatr Surg 2019;54(8): 1539–45.
[15] Cote CJ, Zaslavsky A, Downes JJ, et al. Postoperative apnea in former preterm infants after inguinal herniorrhaphy. A combined analysis. Anesthesiology 1995;82(4):809–22.
[16] Davidson AJ, Morton NS, Arnup SJ, et al. Apnea after awake regional and general anesthesia in infants. Anesthesiology 2015;123(1):38–54.
[17] Dohms K, Hein M, Rossaint R, et al. Inguinal hernia repair in preterm neonates: is there evidence that spinal or general anaesthesia is the better option regarding intraoperative and postoperative complications? A systematic review and meta-analysis. BMJ Open 2019;9(10):e028728.
[18] Lee SL, Gleason JM, Sydorak RM. A critical review of premature infants with inguinal hernias: optimal timing of repair, incarceration risk, and postoperative apnea. J Pediatr Surg 2011;46(1):217–20.
[19] Khan FA, Zeidan N, Larson SD, et al. Inguinal hernias in premature neonates: exploring optimal timing for repair. Pediatr Surg Int 2018;34(11):1157–61.
[20] Ein SH, Njere I, Ein A. Six thousand three hundred sixty-one pediatric inguinal hernias: a 35-year review. J Pediatr Surg 2006;41(5):980–6.
[21] Erdoğan D, Karaman İ, Aslan MK, et al. Analysis of 3776 pediatric inguinal hernia and hydrocele cases in a tertiary center. J Pediatr Surg 2013;48(8):1767–72.
[22] Erez I, Rathause V, Vacian I, et al. Preoperative ultrasound and intraoperative findings of inguinal hernias in children: a prospective study of 642 children. J Pediatr Surg 2002;37(6):865–8.
[23] Dreuning KMA, Ten Broeke CEM, Twisk JWR, et al. Diagnostic accuracy of preoperative ultrasonography in predicting contralateral inguinal hernia in children: a systematic review and meta-analysis. Eur Radiol 2019;29(2):866–76.
[24] Koski ME, Makari JH, Adams MC, et al. Infant communicating hydroceles—do they need immediate repair or might some clinically resolve? J Pediatr Surg 2010;45(3):590–3.
[25] Hall NJ, Ron O, Eaton S, et al. Surgery for hydrocele in children—an avoidable excess? J Pediatr Surg 2011;46(12):2401–5.
[26] Stylianos S, Jacir NN, Harris BH. Incarceration of inguinal hernia in infants prior to elective repair. J Pediatr Surg 1993;28(4):582–3.
[27] Chan YY, Durbin-Johnson B, Kurzrock EA. Pediatric inguinal and scrotal surgery - Practice patterns in U.S. academic centers. J Pediatr Surg 2016;51(11):1786–90.

[28] Ravi K, Hamer DB. Surgical treatment of inguinal herniae in children. Hernia 2003;7(3): 137–40.
[29] Levitt MA, Ferraraccio D, Arbesman MC, et al. Variability of inguinal hernia surgical technique: a survey of North American pediatric surgeons. J Pediatr Surg 2002;37(5):745–51.
[30] Ibrahim M, Ladan MA, Abdussalam US, et al. Open inguinal herniotomy: analysis of variations. Afr J Paediatr Surg 2015;12(2):131–5.
[31] Ostlie DJ, Ponsky TA. Technical options of the laparoscopic pediatric inguinal hernia repair. J Laparoendosc Adv Surg Tech A 2014;24(3):194–8.
[32] Eaton S, Hoellwarth M, Puri P, et al. Management of pediatric inguinal hernias in the era of laparoscopy: results of an international survey. Eur J Pediatr Surg 2013;24(01):009–13.
[33] Esposito C, Escolino M, Turra F, et al. Current concepts in the management of inguinal hernia and hydrocele in pediatric patients in laparoscopic era. Semin Pediatr Surg 2016;25(4): 232–40.
[34] Olesen CS, Andresen K, Oberg S, et al. Laparoscopic versus open repair of groin hernias in children: a systematic review and meta-analysis. Surg Endosc 2019;33(7): 2050–60.
[35] Dreuning K, Maat S, Twisk J, et al. Laparoscopic versus open pediatric inguinal hernia repair: state-of-the-art comparison and future perspectives from a meta-analysis. Surg Endosc 2019;33(10):3177–91.
[36] Jarboe MD. Ultrasound-guided inguinal hernia repair. American Pediatric Surgical Association Annual Meeting; Boston, MA, May 19–22, 2019.
[37] Rothenberg RE, Barnett T. Bilateral herniotomy in infants and children. Surgery 1955;37(6): 947–50.
[38] Burgmeier C, Dreyhaupt J, Schier F. Gender-related differences of inguinal hernia and asymptomatic patent processus vaginalis in term and preterm infants. J Pediatr Surg 2015;50(3):478–80.
[39] Weaver KL, Poola AS, Gould JL, et al. The risk of developing a symptomatic inguinal hernia in children with an asymptomatic patent processus vaginalis. J Pediatr Surg 2017;52(1): 60–4.
[40] Wenk K, Sick B, Sasse T, et al. Incidence of metachronous contralateral inguinal hernias in children following unilateral repair - A meta-analysis of prospective studies. J Pediatr Surg 2015;50(12):2147–54.
[41] Feng S, Zhao L, Liao Z, et al. Open versus laparoscopic inguinal herniotomy in children: a systematic review and meta-analysis focusing on postoperative complications. Surg Laparosc Endosc Percutan Tech 2015;25(4):275–80.
[42] Weber TR. Umbilical and other abdominal wall hernias. 6th edition. Elsevier Saunders; 2014.
[43] Zens T, Nichol PF, Cartmill R, et al. Management of asymptomatic pediatric umbilical hernias: a systematic review. J Pediatr Surg 2017;52(11):1723–31.
[44] Wang X, Xu Z, Miao C-H. Current clinical evidence on the effect of general anesthesia on neurodevelopment in children: an updated systematic review with meta-regression. PLoS One 2014;9(1):e85760.
[45] Glatz P, Sandin RH, Pedersen NL, et al. Association of anesthesia and surgery during childhood with long-term academic performance. JAMA Pediatr 2017;171(1):e163470.
[46] Mamie C, Habre W, Delhumeau C, et al. Incidence and risk factors of perioperative respiratory adverse events in children undergoing elective surgery. Paediatr Anaesth 2004;14(3):218–24.
[47] Zendejas B, Kuchena A, Onkendi EO, et al. Fifty-three–year experience with pediatric umbilical hernia repairs. J Pediatr Surg 2011;46(11):2151–6.
[48] Coats RD, Helikson MA, Burd RS. Presentation and management of epigastric hernias in children. J Pediatr Surg 2000;35(12):1754–6.

[49] Ralls MW, Gadepalli S, Hirschl RB, et al. Ultrasound-Guided Epigastric Hernia Repair. American Pediatric Surgical Association Annual Meeting; Boston, MA, May 19–22, 2019.
[50] Fonkalsrud EW. Femoral and direct inguinal hernias in infants and children. JAMA 1965;192(7):597.
[51] Schier F, Klizaite J. Rare inguinal hernia forms in children. Pediatr Surg Int 2004;20(10): 748–52.
[52] Kelly KB, Ponsky TA. Pediatric abdominal wall defects. Surg Clin North Am 2013;93(5): 1255–67.

Advances in Pediatrics 67 (2020) 145–169

ADVANCES IN PEDIATRICS

Surgical Pulmonary and Pleural Diseases in Children

Lung Malformations, Empyema, and Spontaneous Pneumothorax

Shaun M. Kunisaki, MD, MSc[a,*], Charles M. Leys, MD, MSCI[b]

[a]Division of General Pediatric Surgery, Johns Hopkins Children's Center, Johns Hopkins University, Johns Hopkins University School of Medicine, 1800 Orleans Street, Suite 7353, Baltimore, MD 21287, USA; [b]Division of Pediatric Surgery, University of Wisconsin School of Medicine and Public Health, American Family Children's Hospital, 600 Highland Avenue, H4/740 CSC, Madison, WI 53792-7375, USA

Keywords

- Congenital lung malformations • Congenital pulmonary airway malformations • Bronchopulmonary sequestrations • Parapneumonic effusion • Empyema • Intrapleural fibrinolysis • Spontaneous pneumothorax • Simple aspiration

Key points

- There have been many advances in the management of lung malformations, including enhanced prenatal risk stratification by ultrasound, increasing use of maternal steroids in large fetal lesions, and the widespread adoption of minimally invasive surgical techniques for elective resection.
- Contemporary management of pediatric empyema includes the important diagnostic role of chest ultrasound as well as the emergence of percutaneous chest tube and intrapleural fibrinolysis as the treatment of choice at many centers.
- Primary spontaneous pneumothorax is associated with high recurrence rates after nonoperative management and variability in practice patterns. Minimally invasive approaches and a movement toward earlier surgical intervention may shorten hospitalization, decrease recurrence rates, and reduce the burden of this disease.

*Corresponding author. *E-mail address:* skunisa1@jhmi.edu

https://doi.org/10.1016/j.yapd.2020.03.006
0065-3101/20/

CONGENITAL LUNG MALFORMATIONS

Introduction

Congenital lung malformations are a family of pulmonary lesions that include congenital pulmonary airway malformations (CPAMs), bronchopulmonary sequestrations (BPS), bronchogenic cysts, and congenital lobar emphysema (Fig. 1). Although large-scale, population-based studies on their incidence have not been reported, the incidence of these masses may be as high as 1 in 2500 live births [1,2] because of the widespread use of fetal ultrasound screening. In addition, ongoing improvements in the resolution and enhanced sensitivity of the anatomic survey are contributing to the antenatal detection of smaller masses that do not cause mass effect within the chest.

Lung malformations seem to be sporadic without any association with maternal factors, such as age, smoking status, ethnicity, or parity. Although these lesions are not associated with karyotype anomalies, approximately 5% to 10% of fetuses with a lung malformation will have another type of other concomitant major anomaly [3,4].

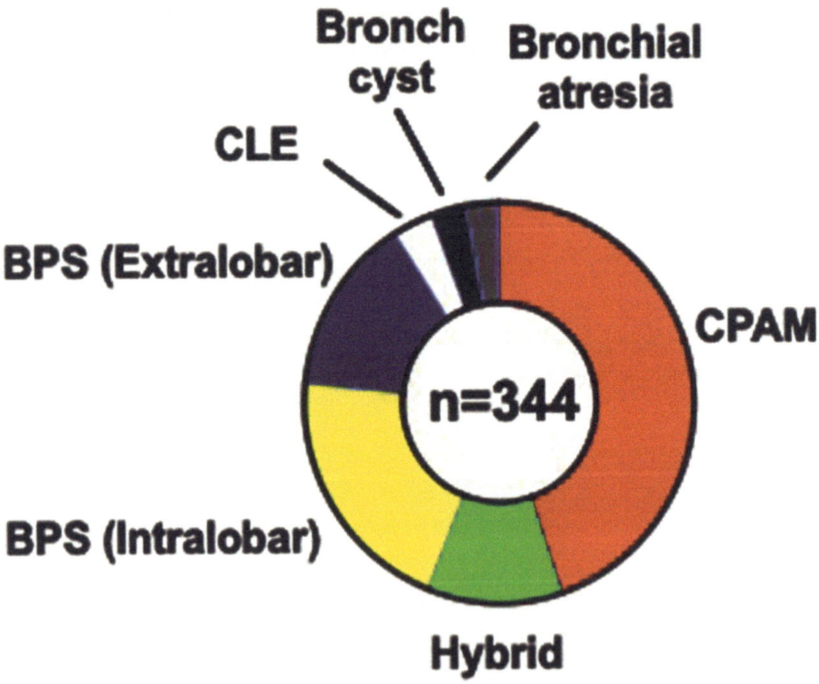

Fig. 1. Donut graph of the relative distribution of congenital lung malformations collected from a multicenter research collaborative [4]. (*Data from* Kunisaki SM, Saito JM, Fallat ME, et al. Development of a multi-institutional registry for children with operative congenital lung malformations. *J Pediatr Surg*. 2019.)

Types of lung malformations

CPAMs (formerly referred to as congenital cystic adenomatoid malformations [CCAM]) are the most common of all lung malformations (Fig. 2) [4]. Stocker's original classification scheme described 3 types of lesions–type I were macrocystic, type II were mixed, and type III were solid/microcystic [5]. However, the nomenclature for these malformations has been revised, and there are now 5 different types, defined by Arabic numerals (0–4) according to relative location of the malformation in relationship to the main airways [6]. The more generic term, CPAMs, as opposed to CCAMs, has been adopted by pathologists in part because microscopic evaluation of resected specimens often revealed that many of these lesions were neither cystic nor adenomatoid. Several gene mutations have been described, but there are currently no modifiable genes identified for the purposes of diagnosis and treatment.

Despite their heterogeneity, all CPAMs are benign and tend to show evidence of aberrant pulmonary morphogenesis corresponding to the pseudoglandular phase of lung development. Transient fetal bronchial obstruction may be an inciting event in disease pathogenesis [7,8]. The hallmark microscopic features of CPAMs include hamartomas as well as an overgrowth of terminal bronchioles. However, in contrast to other lesions, such as BPS and bronchogenic cysts, CPAMs classically communicate directly with normal lung tissue via the bronchial airways. CPAMs do not contain normal alveoli, and therefore function poorly with respect to gas exchange. Larger lesions are known to compromise function of adjacent normal lung tissue because of mass effect. CPAMs tend to involve both lungs at equal rates but are usually

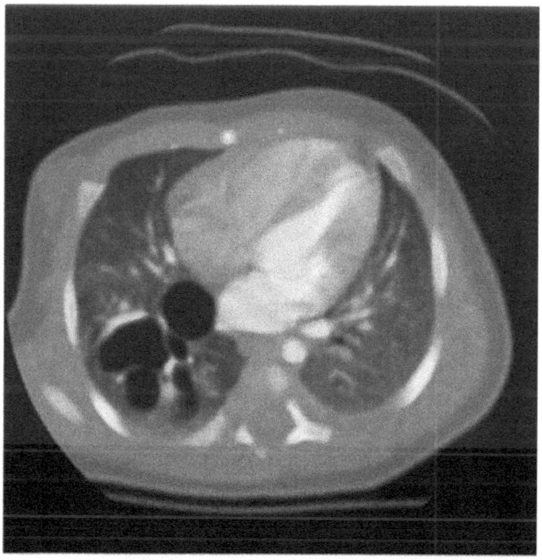

Fig. 2. Axial section from a chest CT scan demonstrating a right lower lobe congenital pulmonary airway malformation in an asymptomatic infant.

unilateral and located in one of the lower lobes in approximately 75% of cases [4].

By definition, the vascular supply of CPAMs is derived from the pulmonary circulation (ie, pulmonary arteries and pulmonary veins). Nevertheless, mixed/hybrid lesions containing components of an intralobar BPS are quite common. These mixed CPAM/BPS masses typically drain into the pulmonary veins but will be supplied by both pulmonary arteries and systemic feeding vessels [9]. The existence of mixed/hybrid lesions supports the notion of a spectrum of lung anomalies with a common disease pathogenesis [8].

The second most common lung malformation is BPS. Because BPS shares many similarities to CPAM, the 2 disease entities are often confused. Both BPS and CPAM have a predisposition to involve the lower lobes and largely contain nonfunctioning tissue and can compromise adjacent lung function by mass effect. Up to 25% of resected lung lesions will have CPAM histology but also have a systemic arterial blood supply (ie, hybrid lesions) [10]. However, as implied by its name, BPS can be distinguished from CPAM based on its lack of communication (sequestration) with respect to the native airways. As a result, BPS lesions are nonaerated pulmonary structures but have potential for collateral ventilation from the adjacent normal lung via the pores of Kohn.

For diagnostic purposes, the presence of a systemic, as opposed to pulmonary, blood vessel is pathognomonic for BPS [11]. The systemic arterial vessels typically arise from the lower thoracic or upper abdominal aorta (Fig. 3), although other origins have also been described (eg, gastric, splenic). Because of its systemic vasculature, large BPS lesions have the unique ability to steal blood flow from other organs, potentially leading to cardiac overload and heart failure over time. BPS lesions are classified anatomically as either intralobar (75%) or extralobar (25%) [4]. Intralobar sequestrations typically involve one of the lower lobes and are entirely invested within the visceral pleura. Because of their close proximity with aerated lung, intralobar variants are predisposed

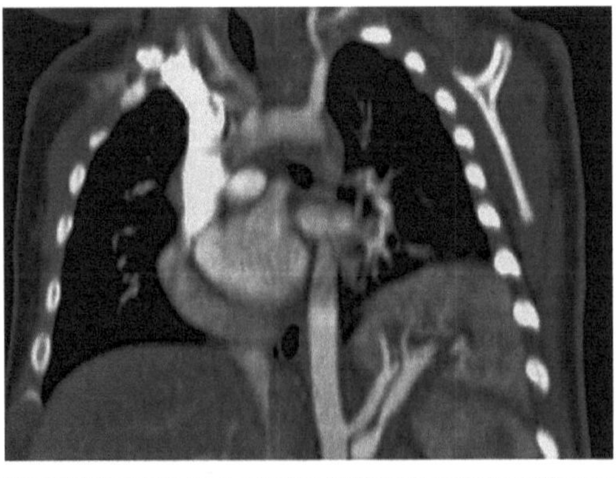

Fig. 3. Coronal section from a chest CT scan illustrating the systemic blood supply associated with a left lower lobe bronchopulmonary sequestration.

to bacterial seeding with subsequent pneumonia. In contrast, extralobar sequestrations are accessory lobes that usually have systemic venous drainage as well as their own pleural covering that is completely separate from normal lung parenchyma. Extralobar variants are therefore less likely to become infected.

Bronchogenic cysts represent a third type of lung malformation. These unilocular masses, which are rare in most major series [4], are thought to represent foregut malformations derived from anomalous budding of the tracheobronchial tree and failure of recanalization during the embryonic stage of lung development [12]. Bronchogenic cysts can sometimes be difficult to distinguish from CPAMs or other duplication cysts based on ultrasound alone. However, in contrast to CPAMs and BPS lesions, bronchogenic cysts are usually paratracheal or adjacent to one of the mainstem bronchi. These lesions tend to be centrally located within the mediastinum and cause problems by way of airway compression with or without distal lung hyperinflation. Another differentiating feature of bronchogenic cysts is their pathology. Bronchogenic cysts contain cartilaginous elements and are lined with ciliated mucus-secreting columnar epithelium that can fill the cyst with mucinous secretions over time. It is thus not surprising that bronchogenic cysts tend to enlarge over time and are susceptible to abscess formation.

Congenital lobar emphysema (CLE) is the fourth type of lung malformation. These lesions are a well-described cause of respiratory distress in neonatal intensive care units but are uncommonly diagnosed in the prenatal period [13]. CLEs are often isoechoic on fetal ultrasound, and many are not associated with significant mediastinal shift until after birth. The term, emphysema, is actually a misnomer since there is no pathologic evidence of lung destruction. Instead, the lobe affected by CLE is susceptible toward overinflation during respiration from a variety of diverse causes, ranging from intrinsic bronchial obstruction, bronchomalacia, extrinsic bronchial obstruction, and polyalveolar lobe [14]. As in CPAMs, transient fetal bronchial obstruction may be important in the disease pathogenesis of CLEs [8]. On fetal ultrasound, the affected lobe may appear opaque or have reticular shadowing with mediastinal shift. There may be little or no change in lung volume, and cysts will be absent. The lack of a systemic vascular supply will rule out BPS.

The end result clinically in most cases of CLE is progressive air trapping with subsequent mediastinal shift and profound respiratory compromise in neonates (Fig. 4). The left upper lobe, sometimes with sparing of the lingual, and the right middle lobe are most commonly affected by CLE. Recently, asymptomatic cases of CLE that involve only segmental portions of a lobe have been appreciated [15]. These lesions may reveal mild bronchial ectasia and are sometimes classified pathologically within the bronchial atresia spectrum. There is no widespread consensus on whether to electively resect asymptomatic CLE.

Prenatal management of lung malformations

More than 70% of lung lesions are now diagnosed prenatally as part of the fetal anatomic surgery (Fig. 5). Recently, numerous studies have shown that lesion

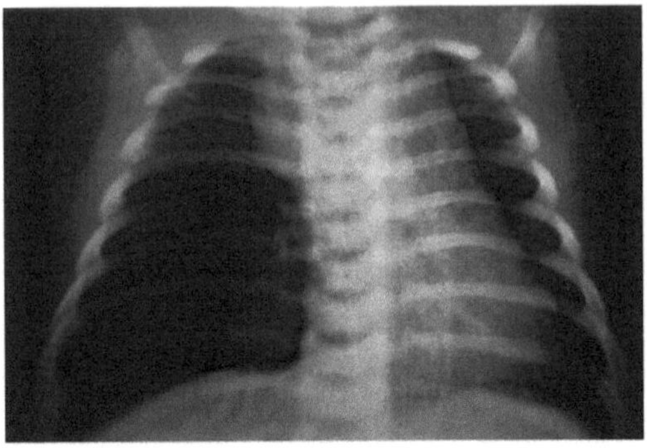

Fig. 4. Anteroposterior chest radiograph showing right middle lobe hyperinflation and mediastinal shift in a neonate secondary to congenital lobar emphysema.

size, rather than malformation type, is most predictive of perinatal outcome, defined broadly based on hydrops, symptomatic disease at birth, and need for subsequent surgery in the neonatal period [3,16–18]. The most common metric for lesion size is the CPAM volume ratio (CVR), which measures the 3D size of the lesion relative to the fetal head circumference [19]. The CVR formula is shown below:

$$\frac{width \times depth \times length \times 0.52}{head\ circumference} = CVR$$

The measurement of the CVR is relatively straightforward, reproducible, and can be performed easily using 2D ultrasound technology based on

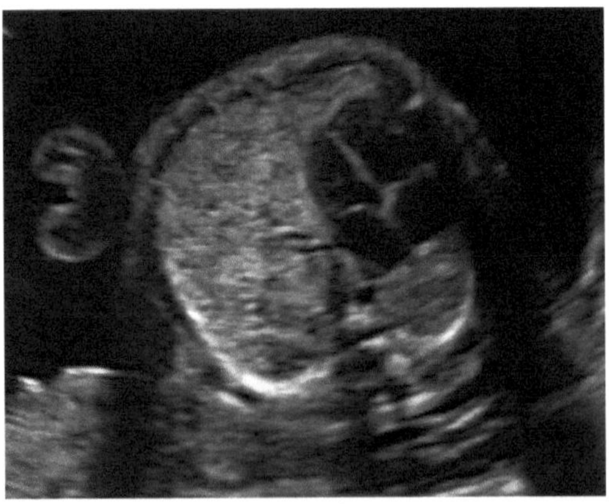

Fig. 5. Axial view of the fetal chest by ultrasound demonstrating a large microcystic lung mass with mass effect on the heart.

transverse and sagittal views. It is also a useful parameter that can be used by different obstetricians as a way to track the size of the lung malformation as the fetus grows over time. Although many maternal-fetal medicine providers have focused on secondary parameters, such as mediastinal shift or polyhydramnios, emerging data suggest that the maximum CVR during pregnancy is the best prognosticator of perinatal outcome [3]. In most fetuses with small-to-moderate sized lung malformations, fetal MRI is probably not cost-effective and adds little additional diagnostic or prognostic information [20]. Given the low incidence of a concomitant cardiac anomalies [4], fetal echocardiography is not mandatory in the prenatal diagnostic evaluation but should be considered on a case-by-case basis.

Most growth patterns in lung malformations can be characterized by initial growth until 26 weeks followed by a subsequent plateau phase and some component of regression after 30 weeks [21]. However, based on fetal lesions identified at the 20-week ultrasound, there are no widely accepted characteristics that can be used to predict which lesions will grow, stabilize, or regress in size. Given the unclear nature of some lesions, it is therefore vital to track their growth trajectory to properly counsel parents and to intervene when appropriate. In rare cases, the mass may actually completely disappear spontaneously (so-called vanishing lesions), although this is usually an artifact given that many lesions often become sonographically isogenic with normal lung parenchyma before term [16,22]. In approximately 40% of sonographically undetectable lesions, a clinically significant lesion is still present using the current gold standard for postnatal imaging, chest computed tomography (CT) [20]. Therefore, when a lesion seems to have vanished, it is prudent to warn parents that both late gestation fetal ultrasound and postnatal chest radiographs (CXRs) have a poor sensitivity for detecting lung malformations, and that the mass might still be present when imaged by CT [16].

One notable advance in the management of prenatal lung malformations is the use of the CVR to guide clinicians on the probability of having asymptomatic disease at birth. Peak CVRs less than 0.9 to 1.0 throughout the pregnancy are reassuring and portend a high likelihood (>90%) of asymptomatic disease at birth (Fig. 6) [3,17]. Even if the lung lesion is small and fetal surgery would be deemed unlikely, consultation with a pediatric surgeon is helpful to establish a relationship with the parents for postnatal follow-up. Most fetuses with small lung malformations can be safely delivered at a local birthing center without substantial neonatal intensive care or pediatric surgical support. A normal vaginal delivery can be performed if a cesarean is not indicated for other maternal or fetal reasons.

However, for large fetal lung malformations, defined as those with persistent/severe mediastinal shift and CVRs consistently well above 1.0, mass effect on native lung tissue can result in impaired lung development with hypoplasia of the adjacent fetal lung [23]. Large masses can also cause mediastinal compression, which often manifests as polyhydramnios secondary to

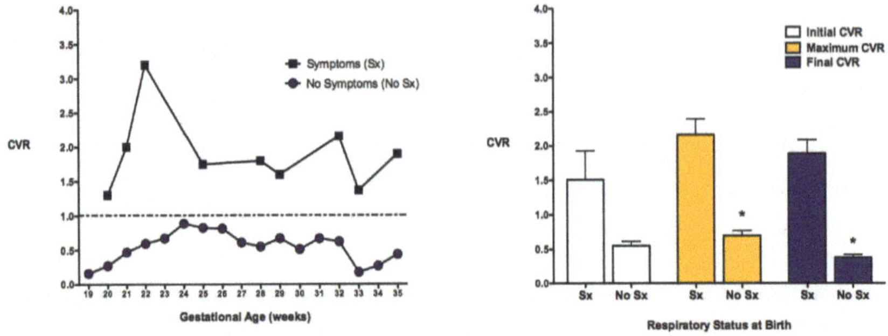

Fig. 6. Association between respiratory symptoms (Sx) at birth and the congenital pulmonary airway malformation volume ratio (CVR) as measured by serial prenatal ultrasound. Line graph of CVR stratified by symptoms (*left*) and vertical bar graph of CVR based on initial, maximum, and final CVR measurements (*right*).* denotes $P<0.05$ compared to symptomatic control.

esophageal obstruction. The most feared complication seen in very large lung malformations is nonimmune hydrops, defined by the presence of 2 or more of the following on prenatal ultrasound: pleural effusion, pericardial effusion, skin edema, or ascites. Placentomegaly and polyhydramnios are also commonly seen. Untreated hydrops from severe mediastinal compression compromise cardiac venous return and ultimately lead to in utero heart failure [24,25]. Fortunately, hydrops is a relatively rare event, occurring in less than 10% of fetuses based on recent reports using multi-institutional data [13]. In the seminal paper correlating the CVR and hydrops, an initial CVR greater than 1.6 identifies a subgroup of fetuses at increased hydrops risk [19].

Over the past decade, another significant advance in the prenatal care of large CPAMs has been the widespread adoption of maternal steroids as the standard of care in the setting of hydrops or impending hydrops [4,26]. The true effectiveness of maternal steroids for large CPAMs remains controversial, but the relatively low maternal-fetal risk profile precludes the ability to study the impact of steroids in a randomized trial. Investigators have speculated that steroids may abrogate aberrant mesenchymal proliferation within the abnormal lung, thereby facilitating the transition from the canalicular to the saccular stage of development [27]. High success rates (80%–90% response) have been reported with maternal steroids use by multiple groups when administered before 26 weeks gestation [27,28]. Anecdotally, the introduction of steroids over the last decade has also been associated with a marked decline in the need to perform open fetal surgery for hydropic fetuses. Thoracoamniotic shunts and ex utero intrapartum treatment procedures are also rarely performed as second-line therapy, constituting less than 5% of prenatal cases [27,29–31]. These therapeutic procedures are best managed at a major fetal referral center with established expertise given their high risk for poorer outcomes.

Postnatal management of lung malformations

Symptomatic neonates constitute approximately 10% of prenatally diagnosed lung malformations and can be predicted based on CVR [3]. In the presence of respiratory compromise, CXRs should be performed immediately to assess for degree of mediastinal shift and to rule out an associated pneumothorax. Additional imaging modalities in larger lung malformations may include an echocardiogram to rule out congenital heart disease and to evaluate for right heart failure and pulmonary hypertension. The vast majority of neonates with symptomatic lung malformations can be definitively treated by thoracotomy and lobectomy [32]. A preoperative CT scan is ideal in most cases since a systemic feeding vessel may be present, regardless of negative findings from prenatal ultrasound [20]. Rarely, a thoracotomy may be required on an emergent basis, particularly in CLE lesions, because of rapid and progressive air trapping exacerbated by positive pressure ventilation. Fortunately, the need for extracorporeal membrane oxygenation (ECMO) to help support these children postoperatively remains relatively uncommon [4,33].

Asymptomatic patients typically have CVRs less than 0.9 to 1.0 and constitute up to 90% of patients with a prenatally diagnosed lung lesion [3,17]. These children have an excellent prognosis and, if desired, can be discharged based on established well-baby guidelines. However, before discharge, CXRs can be helpful as a baseline study for subsequent imaging. It is also important to realize that radiographs often appear normal unless there is an associated mediastinal shift. In several studies, the estimated sensitivity for detecting a lung malformation lesion is only between 50% and 80% [4,34]. Therefore, one can never rule out a congenital lung mass based on radiographs alone.

Follow-up with a pediatric surgeon at between 4 and 12 weeks of age is recommended in all asymptomatic cases. During that time, the child should also undergo a chest CT scan [20]. In infants, obtaining adequate cross-sectional images requires intravenous contrast and potentially sedation/general anesthesia.

The decision to prophylactically resect an asymptomatic lung mass is somewhat controversial and is contingent on the type of lung malformation and other factors [35,36]. However, most American pediatric surgeons still favor preemptive resection of CPAM and BPS lesions to avoid known long-term complications, particularly recurrent pneumonia. In general, CPAMs and intralobar BPS are more susceptible to infection, including pulmonary abscesses and pneumonias refractory to antibiotics, because of impaired mucociliary clearance of pathogens. Unfortunately, the true pneumonia risk has not been well defined and ranges from 5% to 86% [36–38]. Malignant degeneration of CPAMs in the long-term is also a well-described entity [39], but the risk is probably quite low (1%–2%). Case reports of pleuropulmonary blastoma (PPB), a malignant lung tumor seen in infants and associated with the DICER1 mutation, have also been observed in lesions that mimic macrocystic CPAMs on CT scan [40,41]. However, most PPB cases are symptomatic, were not prenatally diagnosed, and do not have a systemic blood supply.

Another advance in the care of lung malformations is the role of nonoperative management as an evolving management strategy in selected cases. Some surgeons in the United Kingdom, Europe, and elsewhere have opted to observe asymptomatic lung malformations, particularly those that were prenatally diagnosed and appear to be small CLEs, CPAMs, or extralobar BPS lesions because their natural history is believed to be more benign [36,42]. In a relatively large British study, only 5% of children had symptoms requiring resection at a median follow-up of 5 years [38]. Observation of selected congenital lung malformations seems reasonable but must be balanced against the long-term costs and radiation risks associated with serial imaging. Furthermore, a serious bout of pneumonia within a lung malformation may not be responsive to antibiotics and often requires prolonged hospitalization. The adhesions that form around a previously infected lesion and the major fissure can also make surgical resection more difficult and dangerous [43].

In expert hands, the operative morbidity of an elective lung resection is low [44]. The last decade has seen the widespread adoption of minimally invasive surgical techniques [45], and approximately half of all elective resections are now performed without a thoracotomy (Fig. 7) [4]. Thoracoscopic lobectomy is associated with excellent cosmesis (Fig. 8). Muscle-sparing thoracotomy incisions are also well tolerated from a pain and long-term musculoskeletal morbidity perspective [10]. In most cases, a formal anatomic lobectomy is performed because partial lobectomies (eg, wedge resections, segmentectomies) have an increased potential of leaving behind residual disease. The median hospital length of stay, regardless of operative approach, is approximately 3 days [45]. There is currently no consensus on timing of elective lung surgery [4], but

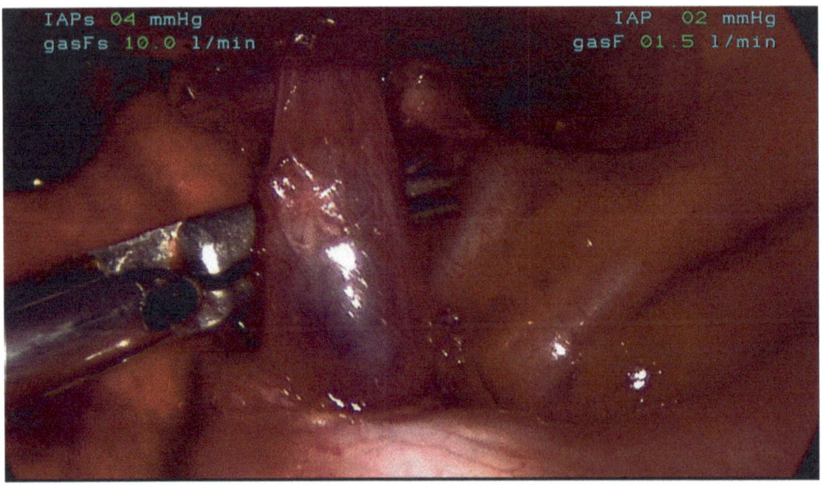

Fig. 7. Intraoperative image showing surgical dissection behind the left inferior pulmonary vein during a thoracoscopic lobectomy performed in an infant.

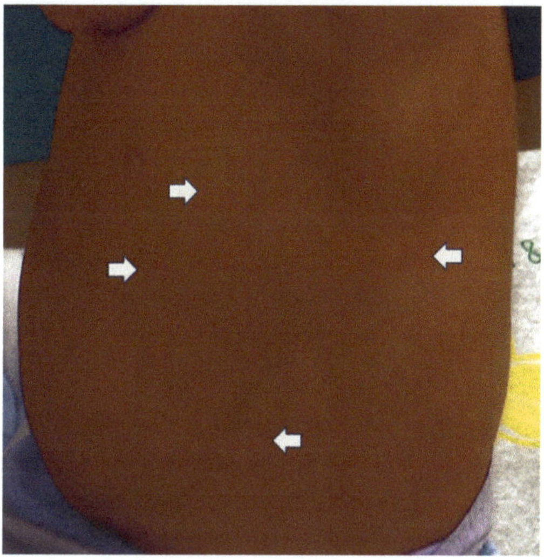

Fig. 8. Typical postoperative appearance of trocar scars (*white arrows*) in a child who underwent thoracoscopic left lower lobectomy at 6 months of age.

many surgeons in North America and Europe prefer to perform lung resections at around 6 months of age before pneumonia occurs and to maximize the potential for compensatory lung growth [10,46,47].

EMPYEMA

Introduction

Empyema, defined as pus within the pleural space, is a well-recognized complication involving 5% to 25% of cases of community-acquired pneumonia, a leading cause of hospitalization in children [48]. Although the overall incidence of empyema has been difficult to quantify, there is no question that its incidence has increased substantially in the past several decades [49]. Children aged 3 to 5 years and prehospitalization ibuprofen use have been implicated as risk factors for empyema [50]. Although most community-acquired pneumonia is viral (eg, respiratory syncytial virus), empyema is most often caused by gram-positive cocci, including *Streptococcus pneumoniae*, *Streptococcus pyogenes* (group A), and *Staphylococcus aureus* [49,51]. *Hemophilus influenza* is a less common pathogen associated with empyema but should still be considered in unvaccinated children. Bilateral empyema secondary to bacterial infection is uncommon.

Empyemas have classically been described along a spectrum defined by 3 stages [52]. During the acute "exudative" phase (stage I, <72 hours), pleural inflammation and increased microvascular permeability lead to the free-flowing accumulation of fluid within the pleural space, resulting in development of a simple parapneumonic effusion. Chemical analysis of the pleural fluid during stage I reveals a pH greater than 7.2 and a lactate dehydrogenase

(LDH) less than 1000 IU. The second stage is the "fibropurulent" phase (stage II, 72 hours to 2 weeks), defined by the development of loculations (often referred to as a loculated parapneumonic effusion) with subsequent development of turbid pleural fluid and pus (empyema) and formation of a fibrinous peel around the visceral pleura. Per the Light criteria, chemical analysis of the pleural fluid in stage II reveals a low pH of less than 7.2, glucose less than 40 mg/dL, and LDH greater than 1000 IU [48]. The pleural fluid white blood cell count should be greater than 10,000 per microliter. After 2 weeks, the infected fluid within the pleural space evolves into a chronic "organizing" phase (stage III), characterized by ongoing deposition of a thick fibrin pleural peel, lung entrapment, and chronic restrictive lung disease.

Diagnosis of empyema

Children with empyema initially present with symptoms typically associated with pneumonia, including cough, dyspnea, tachypnea, anorexia, and/or pyrexia. Severe cases of empyema can manifest clinically as hypoxia, cyanosis, and respiratory distress. Because of pleural involvement, children may also have referred pain to the chest, abdomen, or shoulder. Children with an empyema will often have persistent fevers, oxygen requirement, or leukocytosis despite 48 hours of antibiotic therapy, which often prompts further imaging and surgical consultation on discovery of fluid within the pleural space [48].

Imaging studies can be tremendously helpful in the diagnostic evaluation of empyema. Anteroposterior plain radiographs will usually reveal opacification of the lung field, meniscus sign, obliteration of the costophrenic angle, and possibly mediastinal shift to the contralateral side (Fig. 9). Lateral decubitus plain radiographs can sometimes be helpful to determine whether the pleural

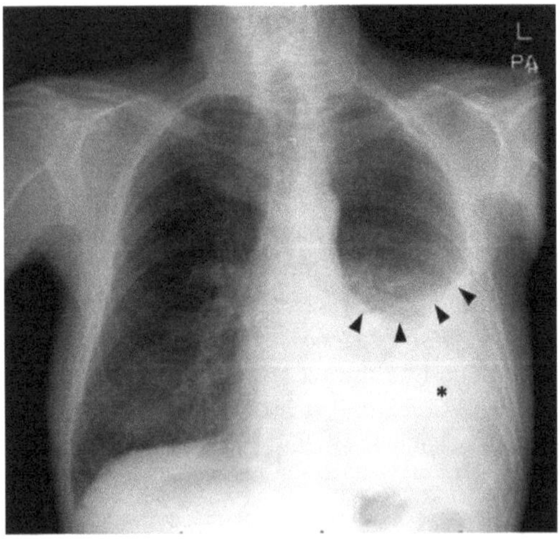

Fig. 9. Anteroposterior chest radiograph demonstrating opacification of the left lower lung field (*asterisk*) with meniscus sign (*arrowheads*) consistent with a moderate left empyema.

fluid layers in a dependent manner, which is more suggestive of a parapneumonic effusion. Another useful imaging modality is chest ultrasound, which has become the favored second study of choice at most children's hospitals. Ultrasound can reliably estimate both the size and characteristics of the effusion. The presence of echogenic material and septations is highly suggestive of an empyema (Fig. 10). Although there is no ionizing radiation with sonographic imaging, it is important to understand that ultrasounds can be limited by operator dependence and poor visualization of aerated lung parenchyma. For these reasons, CT scan continues to be the gold standard that best delineate the thoracic anatomy and remains the best imaging modality of choice to differentiate empyema from other pathologies, including consolidated lung, parenchymal necrosis, intralobar abscess, hemothorax, lung malformations, and cancer, among others. However, because of the potential risks associated with ionizing radiation, chest CT scans for suspected empyema should be reserved for equivocal findings by ultrasound that may affect management recommendations [48].

Both the increasing role of imaging and need for sedation with pediatric procedures has made routine diagnostic thoracentesis less useful in most pediatric cases of suspected empyema [48]. Because most children have already received antibiotics for at least 48 hours, the pleural fluid Gram stain and cultures may not be informative. The role of molecular-based testing of the pleural fluid is evolving but remains unclear [53], and biochemical analyses of the fluid are rarely helpful in the decision-making treatment algorithm of empyema by the surgeon [54]. However, if a malignancy, such as lymphoblastic lymphoma remains in the differential diagnosis based on CT imaging, a thoracentesis is essential, and fluid should be aspirated accordingly for cytologic evaluation.

The key question for many clinicians in the management of a child with a large parapneumonic effusion or empyema is whether the patient's condition

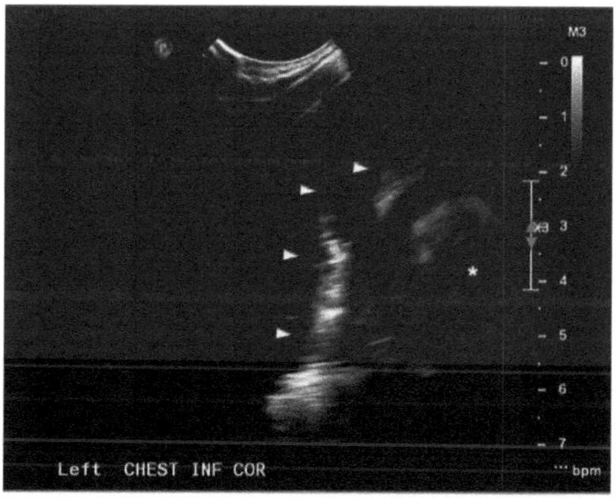

Fig. 10. Representative sonographic view of the left lower chest showing pleural fluid (*left*) with septations (*arrowheads*) and consolidated lung (*asterisk*).

will improve by addressing the pleural disease with a chest tube or other therapeutic intervention. In many cases, the answer is obvious, but in others, the amount of pleural fluid seems unimpressive compared with the degree of intraparenchymal disease. In the latter cases where there may be extensive consolidation, intraparenchymal necrosis, or lung abscess, continued aggressive medical management without surgical intervention may be the most prudent course of action.

Management of empyema

In addition to respiratory support, antipyretics, and analgesia, medical treatment of the underlying pneumonia with intravenous broad-spectrum antibiotics is critical. Depending on institution-specific factors, second- or third-generation cephalosporins administrated by intravenous route are often the initial antibiotics of choice. If *S aureus* is suspected based on the presence of pneumatoceles or available microbiology data, vancomycin or clindamycin should be added. When feasible, sputum should be sent for bacterial culture. There is no indication for routine flexible bronchoscopy in the treatment of empyema.

Management with prolonged antibiotics and a chest tube alone was historically recommended for pediatric empyema and may be adequate treatment for those children with limited disease [55]. However, in most children with empyema, such practices merely result in unnecessary delays in appropriate care and increased hospital charges [56]. There is now general consensus among pediatric surgeons that most loculated parapneumonic effusions and empyemas require more aggressive treatment, in the form of either chest drainage with intrapleural fibrinolysis or video-assisted thoracoscopic surgery (VATS) with decortication.

The first major reports on the use of intrapleural fibrinolytic therapy in children were published decades ago [49,57]. In this approach, a percutaneous chest tube (eg, 12 Fr Thal-Quick, Cook Medical, Bloomington, IN, USA) is inserted into the pleural collection using the Seldinger technique under conscious sedation and ultrasound guidance. Chest tube insertion should ideally be performed by a pediatric surgeon or interventional radiologist. Other chest drains, including pigtail catheters, can also be used [58,59], and there is little evidence that large-bore chest drains confer any advantage compared with appropriately placed smaller drains. After the empyema has been drained, a fibrinolytic agent, such as tissue plasminogen activator (tPA, alteplase, Genentech, South San Francision, CA, USA; 4 mg/40 mL saline), is instilled into the chest tube. tPA is a serine protease that assists in fibrin degradation by converting plasminogen to plasmin. In smaller children (<40 kg), weight-based dosing protocols (tPA 0.1 mg/kg) can also be used. The tube is then clamped for at least 1 hour to allow the medication to dwell in the pleural space before connecting the tube to continuous suction. Standard protocols using tPA mandate a total of 3 doses, each given at 24-hour intervals. Contraindications to intrapleural fibrinolysis include bronchopleural fistula, necrotizing pneumonia, and substantial risk for hemorrhage (eg, major coagulopathy, ongoing bleeding on ECMO). For treatment failures after fibrinolytic therapy, which is often defined as persistent pleural disease and failure of clinical response after 4 to 7 days, consideration should be made for chest tube replacement under image guidance plus another round of fibrinolysis versus VATS with decortication (see later discussion), depending on clinical scenario and operative risk.

As an alternative to intrapleural fibrinolysis, VATS continues to embraced by many pediatric surgeons. This operative procedure, which requires full operating room personnel/resources and general endotracheal anesthesia, entails using several 5-mm surgical instruments under direct vision to manually break up pleural loculations and to drain the empyema. Decortication, which involves removing the fibrous rind encasing the entrapped lung, should also be performed in the presence of an organizing pleural rind to help achieve better lung expansion [60]. Drainage of any intralobar lung abscesses is not required and may be associated with increased risk. If a peripheral bronchopleural fistula is present, pneumolysis, chest drainage, and continued antibiotics are usually sufficient. Although uncommon, those fistulae that fail more conservative management strategies may require more complex operative intervention, including additional decortication, muscle flaps, and other maneuvers [61]. A chest tube is left in the pleural space at the end of the procedure to collect residual fluid and to help re-expand the lung postoperatively. Several studies have demonstrated that VATS is well tolerated and is a more effective treatment strategy for empyema when compared with chest tube alone [62,63]. A major contraindication to VATS includes an inability to tolerate the unilateral pneumothorax that is required to visualize the pleural space. This scenario is common in the setting of profound respiratory failure with extensive parenchymal disease. In children with extensive stage III disease, where entering the chest with multiple trocars may be not be feasible, a thoracotomy incision may be therefore required to facilitate evacuation of the empyema [64].

Although VATS was the preferred treatment of empyema based on several case series [62,64,65], the pendulum has swung in the last decade in favor of intrapleural fibrinolytic therapy treatment as the first-line treatment option [66,67]. This paradigm shift is based on evidence from at least 3 randomized trials conducted in the United States and in Europe [68–70], all demonstrating the equivalence of intrapleural fibrinolytic therapy when compared with VATS for the management of empyema. Most of these studies showed no difference in outcomes between intrapleural fibrinolysis and VATS, based on hospital length of stay, oxygen requirement, febrile state, and analgesia dosing. The treatment failure rate of the 2 procedures was also similar (10%–15%).

Proponents of intrapleural fibrinolysis also cite slightly lower complication rates, but the relatively small sample size of these studies raises concern about whether they are sufficiently powered to adequately address that issue. Intrapleural fibrinolysis has also been associated with a 25% to 50% reduction in hospital charges in some studies [71], but local institutional factors, including access to the sedation facilities as well as the relative cost/availability of operating rooms, should be considered [72]. Moreover, if the child is undergoing a general anesthetic for chest drain insertion anyway, the threshold for combining the procedure with VATS seems compelling to many providers. The pharmacy cost for 3 doses of tPA in the United States is variable but may approach $1000 [73]. In practice, it is unlikely that any one method of treatment will be superior to the other when applied to a heterogenous group of children with empyema.

Clinical improvement (eg, weaning of oxygen support) is expected over the next 3 to 4 days in children with empyema after either intrapleural fibrinolysis or VATS. The utility of daily CXRs is controversial since radiologic improvement often lags behind clinical response. Chest drains are maintained on continuous suction (eg, 20 cm H_2O) and should be managed by pediatric surgeons to minimize tube-related complications, such as occlusion by fibrous clots and other debris. Routine saline flushes of the chest tube may be required to maintain patency. The drain can typically be removed if there is no air leak and output is less than 1 to 2 mL/kg over a 24-hour period. The median length of stay postintervention is typically between 5 and 10 days [74]. Mortality rates are very low and usually related to associated comorbidities. Antibiotics are typically continued with oral agents for a total course of 2 to 4 weeks. Most children make a complete recovery and have no long-term sequelae from the empyema based on exercise tolerance and pulmonary function testing [75].

Ongoing research topics in pediatric empyema largely revolve around patient-centered outcomes and ongoing refinements in diagnosis and treatment [76]. For example, it is unclear which subgroups of children with empyemas are more likely to benefit from one approach compared with the other [77]. Development and optimization of intrapleural fibrinolysis protocols are also active areas of inquiry. The added benefit of using additional intrapleural agents, such as dornase alfa (rhDNase), in conjunction with tPA has been demonstrated in randomized trial in adults [78], and a multicenter Canadian study using 5 mg of rhDNase in children is forthcoming [79].

PRIMARY SPONTANEOUS PNEUMOTHORAX

Presentation

Pneumothorax is defined as air in the pleural space and results in collapse of the ipsilateral lung of varying degrees. Primary spontaneous pneumothorax (PSP) refers to a pneumothorax that occurs without any known inciting event, such as trauma or an invasive procedure, and is not secondary to an underlying pulmonary disease, such as asthma, cystic fibrosis, interstitial lung disease, connective tissue disorder, congenital lung lesion, or malignancy. The underlying cause of PSP is often previously undiagnosed blebs, abnormal cyst-like lesions on the lung surface, usually near the apex, that can rupture and leak air from the lung into the pleural space (Fig. 11). PSP primarily occurs in adolescents and young adults, with an estimated incidence in children of 3.4 per 100,000 and a 4:1 male/female ratio [80]. The typical patient has a tall, thin body habitus. The most common presenting symptoms are acute onset chest

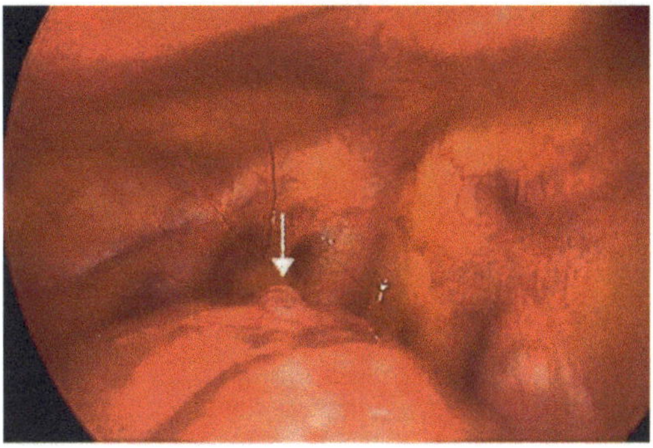

Fig. 11. Thoracoscopic view of apical bleb before wedge resection. White arrow refer to apical bleb.

pain and mild shortness of breath. Some patients may have had symptoms for several days before seeking medical attention and may report previous episodes that resolved spontaneously. Factors that predispose a patient to bleb rupture include any activity that increases intrathoracic or airway pressures, such as forceful coughing, weightlifting, or playing a brass musical instrument, such as horn or trumpet.

For diagnosis, history and physical exam are important to exclude other potential underlying causes. Breath sounds may be decreased on the affected side, although they may be normal if the pneumothorax is small. Tension pneumothorax physiology is quite rare, but it is important to recognize in patients presenting with signs such as tachycardia, hypotension, hypoxia, and tracheal deviation to the contralateral side. Once suspected, the diagnosis of PSP is easily confirmed with just a plain upright posteroanterior CXR, which will show a pneumothorax and occasionally may even show unilateral or bilateral blebs (Fig. 12A). A CT scan is usually not necessary, and evidence suggests that it is not generally helpful, unless it is needed to definitively rule out other causes [81,82]. Some surgeons use a CT scan in cases of recurrent disease or to look for location or bilaterality of the blebs, which could alter the surgical plan, although thoracoscopic visualization is more sensitive than CT scan for identifying blebs [81,82].

Management

The optimal initial management of PSP in children remains unclear and evidence-based guidelines are lacking, resulting in significant practice variability. In general, there is good consensus that a small PSP that is not recurrent in a stable, minimally symptomatic patient can be observed, whereas a moderate to large or severely symptomatic PSP will require either chest tube placement or simple aspiration to evacuate the pneumothorax [83–85]. Surgical intervention has traditionally been reserved for recurrent disease, bilateral disease, or failure of chest tube management due to persistent air leak or

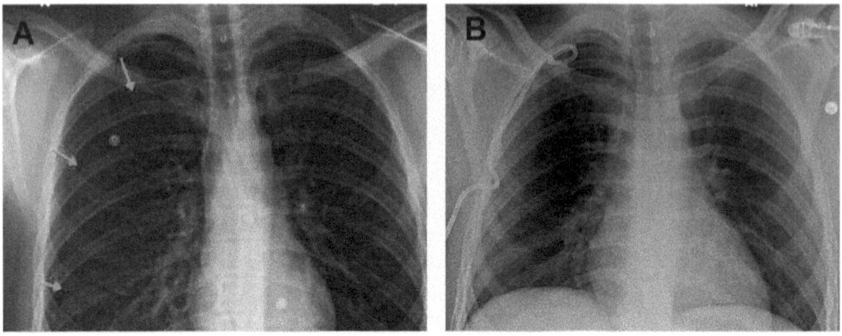

Fig. 12. (*A*) Anteroposterior chest radiograph demonstrating a right pneumothorax. (*B*) Anteroposterior chest radiograph after right pigtail catheter placement. Blue arrows refer to visible pleural border consistent with the pneumothorax.

inadequate lung expansion. Tension physiology should be treated immediately with a large-bore needle or angiocatheter inserted at the second intercostal space in the mid-clavicular line anteriorly to evacuate the pneumothorax, usually followed by chest tube placement or surgery.

Observation is appropriate initial management for a first-episode, small pneumothorax without dyspnea, and can result in resolution in up to 80% of small PSP [83,84]. Defining what constitutes a small pneumothorax can be a challenge, however, especially in children of varying age and size, and existing guidelines for adults are not consistent. A consensus statement published by the American College of Chest Physicians (ACCP) suggests observation for PSP with less than 3 cm distance between the apex of the lung and the top of the pleural space on plain anteroposterior CXR [85]. The 2010 British Thoracic Society (BTS) guidelines suggest using the threshold of 2 cm distance between the lung and the chest wall laterally at the level of the hilum [84]. Both techniques can underestimate the size of the pneumothorax, however, so another useful strategy estimates pneumothorax size as a percentage of thoracic volume, often calculated with the Light method and using a 15% threshold to define small versus large [83]. Observation can be performed with or without monitoring or supplemental oxygen, which may help speed resolution, and either as inpatient or in the emergency department for 3 to 6 hours. If the patient remains minimally symptomatic and pneumothorax size is stable on repeat CXR after a period of observation, the patient can be discharged home with close outpatient follow-up and instruction on symptoms that should prompt immediate return [85]. Such outpatient management may not be appropriate for patients who live far from the medical center or when proper follow-up cannot be ensured.

A first-episode PSP that is moderate to large in size or associated with dyspnea or significant pain necessitates an intervention to evacuate the pneumothorax. This is most often accomplished with a nonoperative approach, using either a simple aspiration procedure (ie, thoracentesis) or percutaneous insertion of a small-bore chest tube or catheter (tube thoracostomy). Simple aspiration can be performed as an outpatient procedure and is the recommended next step in the 2010 BTS guidelines, reserving chest tube management for failure of aspiration [84]. In contrast, the 2001 ACCP Delphi consensus statement recommends chest tube placement as the first-line intervention, which is the most common approach for North American Pediatric Surgeons, despite that fact that this approach can be associated with prolonged hospitalization [85,86]. Tube thoracostomy can be performed with a small 8 to 12 French soft pigtail catheter with Seldinger technique, since the tube only needs to evacuate air (Fig. 12B). If a patient with a chest tube demonstrates continued air leak and lack of PSP resolution after 4 days of chest tube management, surgery should be considered [85].

Both nonoperative techniques can resolve a PSP in up to 80% to 90% of patients, but unfortunately recurrence of PSP after successful nonoperative management is quite high at 40% to 60% [87–95]. Two recent studies found that 63% to 80% of patients with PSP ultimately end up requiring surgery for definitive treatment [88,90]. In light of these poor outcomes with nonoperative management, its association with sometimes frustratingly long hospitalizations, and now widespread availability of minimally invasive thoracic surgical techniques (VATS), some surgeons have started to offer primary VATS as the initial intervention for first-episode PSP [88,93,94]. However, studies have found that primary VATS is not a cost-effective strategy and potentially exposes some patients to the risk of surgery who may not have needed it [90,92]. Recent evidence suggests that a decision to proceed to earlier surgery may shorten hospital stay and decrease recurrence rates, but early predictors are needed to determine which patients are likely to fail nonoperative management [88,90,96]. A more recent pilot study found that simple aspiration may be useful as such a predictor, as 83% of patients who failed aspiration ultimately required surgery due to either persistent air leak or recurrence [97]. The authors proposed a management algorithm whereby surgery would be the immediate next step after failure of aspiration, thus eliminating the option of chest tube management altogether (Fig. 13).

Surgery is necessary for those who fail less invasive interventions due to either persistent air leak, recurrence of PSP, or the rare instance of bilateral PSP on presentation. The standard surgical approach today uses minimally invasive principles, known commonly as VATS, to identify and remove the bleb(s). This is accomplished with a nonanatomic stapled wedge resection or "blebectomy," usually at the lung apex. Unfortunately, recurrences can occur after VATS as well, with pediatric series reporting 12% to 15% ipsilateral and up to 28% contralateral recurrences [90–92,98]. Bleb formation is believed to be a dynamic process throughout adolescence, so recurrences are most often due to new bleb formation, usually at the apex near the site of prior resection, but can be due to new or previously unrecognized blebs in lower lobes [98]. In an effort to minimize the chance of recurrence after VATS, or to reduce the extent

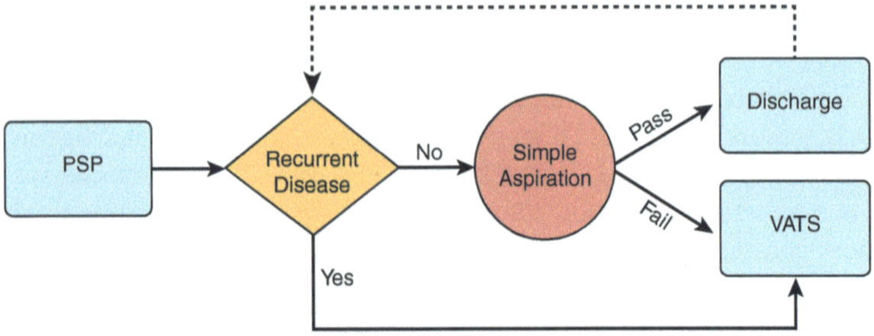

Fig. 13. Proposed PSP management algorithm incorporating simple aspiration to guide decision for operative intervention. (*Adapted from* Leys CM, Hirschl RB, Kohler JE, et al. Changing the Paradigm for Management of Pediatric Primary Spontaneous Pneumothorax: A Simple Aspiration Test Predicts Need for Operation. J Pediatr Surg. 2019 Oct 24; with permission.)

of collapse if a recurrence occurs, blebectomy is often combined with some type of pleurodesis to create adhesions in or obliterate the pleural space. A recent survey found that for a patient's first VATS most North American Pediatric Surgeons perform blebectomy plus mechanical pleurodesis, which involves abrasion of the parietal pleura with a surgical instrument [86]. Pleurodesis may also be performed with pleurectomy, removal of the parietal pleura from the superior portion of the chest cavity, or chemical pleurodesis with agents, such as talc or doxycline placed in the pleural cavity. Studies have been unable to define the optimal surgical technique and wide variability exists in practice, but recent evidence suggests that the addition of chemical pleurodesis at time of blebectomy may be superior to mechanical abrasion [98,99]. Both contralateral and ipsilateral recurrences are most often treated with repeat VATS, although can be treated nonoperatively as well, depending on size, circumstances, and surgeon judgment.

Disclosure

The authors have nothing to disclose.

References

[1] Lima JS, Camargos PA, Aguiar RA, et al. Pre and perinatal aspects of congenital cystic adenomatoid malformation of the lung. J Matern Fetal Neonatal Med 2014;27(3):228–32.
[2] Lau CT, Kan A, Shek N, et al. Is congenital pulmonary airway malformation really a rare disease? Result of a prospective registry with universal antenatal screening program. Pediatr Surg Int 2017;33(1):105–8.
[3] Ehrenberg-Buchner S, Stapf AM, Berman DR, et al. Fetal lung lesions: can we start to breathe easier? Am J Obstet Gynecol 2013;208(2):151.e1-7.
[4] Kunisaki SM, Saito JM, Fallat ME, et al. Development of a multi-institutional registry for children with operative congenital lung malformations. J Pediatr Surg 2019; https://doi.org/10.1016/j.jpedsurg.2019.01.058.
[5] Stocker JT, Madewell JE, Drake RM. Congenital cystic adenomatoid malformation of the lung. Classification and morphologic spectrum. Hum Pathol 1977;8(2):155–71.

[6] Stocker JT. Cystic lung disease in infants and children. Fetal Pediatr Pathol 2009;28(4): 155–84.
[7] Langston C. New concepts in the pathology of congenital lung malformations. Semin Pediatr Surg 2003;12(1):17–37.
[8] Kunisaki SM, Fauza DO, Nemes LP, et al. Bronchial atresia: the hidden pathology within a spectrum of prenatally diagnosed lung masses. J Pediatr Surg 2006;41(1):61–5 [discussion: 61–5].
[9] Cass DL, Crombleholme TM, Howell LJ, et al. Cystic lung lesions with systemic arterial blood supply: a hybrid of congenital cystic adenomatoid malformation and bronchopulmonary sequestration. J Pediatr Surg 1997;32(7):986–90.
[10] Tsai AY, Liechty KW, Hedrick HL, et al. Outcomes after postnatal resection of prenatally diagnosed asymptomatic cystic lung lesions. J Pediatr Surg 2008;43(3):513–7.
[11] Ruano R, Benachi A, Aubry MC, et al. Prenatal diagnosis of pulmonary sequestration using three-dimensional power Doppler ultrasound. Ultrasound Obstet Gynecol 2005;25(2): 128–33.
[12] Fievet L, D'Journo XB, Guys JM, et al. Bronchogenic cyst: best time for surgery? Ann Thorac Surg 2012;94(5):1695–9.
[13] Kunisaki SM, Saito JM, Fallat ME, et al. Current operative management of congenital lobar emphysema in children: a report from the Midwest Pediatric Surgery Consortium. J Pediatr Surg 2019;54(6):1138–42.
[14] Tapper D, Schuster S, McBride J, et al. Polyalveolar lobe: anatomic and physiologic parameters and their relationship to congenital lobar emphysema. J Pediatr Surg 1980;15(6): 931–7.
[15] Mei-Zahav M, Konen O, Manson D, et al. Is congenital lobar emphysema a surgical disease? J Pediatr Surg 2006;41(6):1058–61.
[16] Kunisaki SM, Ehrenberg-Buchner S, Dillman JR, et al. Vanishing fetal lung malformations: prenatal sonographic characteristics and postnatal outcomes. J Pediatr Surg 2015;50(6): 978–82.
[17] Ruchonnet-Metrailler I, Leroy-Terquem E, Stirnemann J, et al. Neonatal outcomes of prenatally diagnosed congenital pulmonary malformations. Pediatrics 2014;133(5):e1285–91.
[18] Girsen AI, Hintz SR, Sammour R, et al. Prediction of neonatal respiratory distress in pregnancies complicated by fetal lung masses. Prenat Diagn 2017;37(3):266–72.
[19] Crombleholme TM, Coleman B, Hedrick H, et al. Cystic adenomatoid malformation volume ratio predicts outcome in prenatally diagnosed cystic adenomatoid malformation of the lung. J Pediatr Surg 2002;37(3):331–8.
[20] Mon RA, Johnson KN, Ladino-Torres M, et al. Diagnostic accuracy of imaging studies in congenital lung malformations. Arch Dis Child Fetal Neonatal Ed 2019;104(4):F372–7.
[21] Macardle CA, Ehrenberg-Buchner S, Smith EA, et al. Surveillance of fetal lung lesions using the congenital pulmonary airway malformation volume ratio: natural history and outcomes. Prenat Diagn 2016;36(3):282–9.
[22] Meizner I, Rosenak D. The vanishing fetal intrathoracic mass: consider an obstructing mucous plug. Ultrasound Obstet Gynecol 1995;5(4):275–7.
[23] Cass DL, Olutoye OO, Cassady CI, et al. Prenatal diagnosis and outcome of fetal lung masses. J Pediatr Surg 2011;46(2):292–8.
[24] Adzick NS. Management of fetal lung lesions. Clin Perinatol 2009;36(2):363–76, x.
[25] Cass DL, Olutoye OO, Ayres NA, et al. Defining hydrops and indications for open fetal surgery for fetuses with lung masses and vascular tumors. J Pediatr Surg 2012;47(1):40–5.
[26] Peranteau WH, Wilson RD, Liechty KW, et al. Effect of maternal betamethasone administration on prenatal congenital cystic adenomatoid malformation growth and fetal survival. Fetal Diagn Ther 2007;22(5):365–71.
[27] Loh KC, Jelin E, Hirose S, et al. Microcystic congenital pulmonary airway malformation with hydrops fetalis: steroids vs open fetal resection. J Pediatr Surg 2012;47(1):36–9.

[28] Morris LM, Lim FY, Livingston JC, et al. High-risk fetal congenital pulmonary airway malformations have a variable response to steroids. J Pediatr Surg 2009;44(1):60–5.
[29] Grethel EJ, Wagner AJ, Clifton MS, et al. Fetal intervention for mass lesions and hydrops improves outcome: a 15-year experience. J Pediatr Surg 2007;42(1):117–23.
[30] Hedrick HL, Flake AW, Crombleholme TM, et al. The ex utero intrapartum therapy procedure for high-risk fetal lung lesions. J Pediatr Surg 2005;40(6):1038–43 [discussion: 1044].
[31] Adzick NS, Harrison MR, Crombleholme TM, et al. Fetal lung lesions: management and outcome. Am J Obstet Gynecol 1998;179(4):884–9.
[32] Johnson KN, Mon RA, Gadepalli SK, et al. Short-term respiratory outcomes of neonates with symptomatic congenital lung malformations. J Pediatr Surg 2019;54(9):1766–70.
[33] Kunisaki SM, Fauza DO, Barnewolt CE, et al. Ex utero intrapartum treatment with placement on extracorporeal membrane oxygenation for fetal thoracic masses. J Pediatr Surg 2007;42(2):420–5.
[34] Calvert JK, Lakhoo K. Antenatally suspected congenital cystic adenomatoid malformation of the lung: postnatal investigation and timing of surgery. J Pediatr Surg 2007;42(2):411–4.
[35] Aziz D, Langer JC, Tuuha SE, et al. Perinatally diagnosed asymptomatic congenital cystic adenomatoid malformation: to resect or not? J Pediatr Surg 2004;39(3):329–34 [discussion: 329–34].
[36] Criss CN, Musili N, Matusko N, et al. Asymptomatic congenital lung malformations: is nonoperative management a viable alternative? J Pediatr Surg 2018;53(6):1092–7.
[37] Wong A, Vieten D, Singh S, et al. Long-term outcome of asymptomatic patients with congenital cystic adenomatoid malformation. Pediatr Surg Int 2009;25(6):479–85.
[38] Ng C, Stanwell J, Burge DM, et al. Conservative management of antenatally diagnosed cystic lung malformations. Arch Dis Child 2014;99(5):432–7.
[39] Casagrande A, Pederiva F. Association between congenital lung malformations and lung tumors in children and adults: a systematic review. J Thorac Oncol 2016;11(11):1837–45.
[40] Miniati DN, Chintagumpala M, Langston C, et al. Prenatal presentation and outcome of children with pleuropulmonary blastoma. J Pediatr Surg 2006;41(1):66–71.
[41] Nasr A, Himidan S, Pastor AC, et al. Is congenital cystic adenomatoid malformation a premalignant lesion for pleuropulmonary blastoma? J Pediatr Surg 2010;45(6):1086–9.
[42] Lo AY, Jones S. Lack of consensus among Canadian pediatric surgeons regarding the management of congenital cystic adenomatoid malformation of the lung. J Pediatr Surg 2008;43(5):797–9.
[43] Durell J, Thakkar H, Gould S, et al. Pathology of asymptomatic, prenatally diagnosed cystic lung malformations. J Pediatr Surg 2016;51(2):231–5.
[44] Rothenberg SS, Kuenzler KA, Middlesworth W, et al. Thoracoscopic lobectomy in infants less than 10 kg with prenatally diagnosed cystic lung disease. J Laparoendosc Adv Surg Tech A 2011;21(2):181–4.
[45] Kunisaki SM, Powelson IA, Haydar B, et al. Thoracoscopic vs open lobectomy in infants and young children with congenital lung malformations. J Am Coll Surg 2014;218(2):261–70.
[46] Conforti A, Aloi I, Trucchi A, et al. Asymptomatic congenital cystic adenomatoid malformation of the lung: is it time to operate? J Thorac Cardiovasc Surg 2009;138(4):826–30.
[47] Jelin EB, O'Hare EM, Jancelewicz T, et al. Optimal timing for elective resection of asymptomatic congenital pulmonary airway malformations. J Pediatr Surg 2018;53(5):1001–5.
[48] Balfour-Lynn IM, Abrahamson E, Cohen G, et al. BTS guidelines for the management of pleural infection in children. Thorax 2005;60(Suppl 1):i1–21.
[49] Byington CL, Spencer LY, Johnson TA, et al. An epidemiological investigation of a sustained high rate of pediatric parapneumonic empyema: risk factors and microbiological associations. Clin Infect Dis 2002;34(4):434–40.
[50] Elemraid MA, Thomas MF, Blain AP, et al. Risk factors for the development of pleural empyema in children. Pediatr Pulmonol 2015;50(7):721–6.

[51] Grijalva CG, Nuorti JP, Zhu Y, et al. Increasing incidence of empyema complicating childhood community-acquired pneumonia in the United States. Clin Infect Dis 2010;50(6): 805–13.
[52] Hamm H, Light RW. Parapneumonic effusion and empyema. Eur Respir J 1997;10(5): 1150–6.
[53] Blaschke AJ, Heyrend C, Byington CL, et al. Molecular analysis improves pathogen identification and epidemiologic study of pediatric parapneumonic empyema. Pediatr Infect Dis J 2011;30(4):289–94.
[54] Becker A, Amantea SL, Fraga JC, et al. Impact of antibiotic therapy on laboratory analysis of parapneumonic pleural fluid in children. J Pediatr Surg 2011;46(3):452–7.
[55] Carter E, Waldhausen J, Zhang W, et al. Management of children with empyema: pleural drainage is not always necessary. Pediatr Pulmonol 2010;45(5):475–80.
[56] Aziz A, Healey JM, Qureshi F, et al. Comparative analysis of chest tube thoracostomy and video-assisted thoracoscopic surgery in empyema and parapneumonic effusion associated with pneumonia in children. Surg Infect (Larchmt) 2008;9(3):317–23.
[57] Rosen H, Nadkarni V, Theroux M, et al. Intrapleural streptokinase as adjunctive treatment for persistent empyema in pediatric patients. Chest 1993;103(4):1190–3.
[58] Pierrepoint MJ, Evans A, Morris SJ, et al. Pigtail catheter drain in the treatment of empyema thoracis. Arch Dis Child 2002;87(4):331–2.
[59] Petel D, Li P, Emil S. Percutaneous pigtail catheter versus tube thoracostomy for pediatric empyema: a comparison of outcomes. Surgery 2013;154(4):655–60 [discussion: 660–51].
[60] Kosloske AM, Cartwright KC. The controversial role of decortication in the management of pediatric empyema. J Thorac Cardiovasc Surg 1988;96(1):166–70.
[61] Hallows MR, Parikh DH. Surgical management of children with pyopneumothorax: serratus anterior digitation flap. J Pediatr Surg 2004;39(7):1122–4.
[62] Cohen G, Hjortdal V, Ricci M, et al. Primary thoracoscopic treatment of empyema in children. J Thorac Cardiovasc Surg 2003;125(1):79–83 [discussion: 83–4].
[63] Avansino JR, Goldman B, Sawin RS, et al. Primary operative versus nonoperative therapy for pediatric empyema: a meta-analysis. Pediatrics 2005;115(6):1652–9.
[64] Klena JW, Cameron BH, Langer JC, et al. Timing of video-assisted thoracoscopic debridement for pediatric empyema. J Am Coll Surg 1998;187(4):404–8.
[65] Grewal H, Jackson RJ, Wagner CW, et al. Early video-assisted thoracic surgery in the management of empyema. Pediatrics 1999;103(5):e63.
[66] Kelly MM, Coller RJ, Kohler JE, et al. Trends in hospital treatment of empyema in children in the United States. J Pediatr 2018;202:245–51.e1.
[67] Dorman RM, Vali K, Rothstein DH. Trends in treatment of infectious parapneumonic effusions in U.S. children's hospitals, 2004-2014. J Pediatr Surg 2016;51(6):885–90.
[68] Sonnappa S, Cohen G, Owens CM, et al. Comparison of urokinase and video-assisted thoracoscopic surgery for treatment of childhood empyema. Am J Respir Crit Care Med 2006;174(2):221–7.
[69] St Peter SD, Tsao K, Spilde TL, et al. Thoracoscopic decortication vs tube thoracostomy with fibrinolysis for empyema in children: a prospective, randomized trial. J Pediatr Surg 2009;44(1):106–11 [discussion: 111].
[70] Marhuenda C, Barcelo C, Fuentes I, et al. Urokinase versus VATS for treatment of empyema: a randomized multicenter clinical trial. Pediatrics 2014;134(5):e1301–7.
[71] Cohen E, Weinstein M, Fisman DN. Cost-effectiveness of competing strategies for the treatment of pediatric empyema. Pediatrics 2008;121(5):e1250–7.
[72] Shah SS, Ten Have TR, Metlay JP. Costs of treating children with complicated pneumonia: a comparison of primary video-assisted thoracoscopic surgery and chest tube placement. Pediatr Pulmonol 2010;45(1):71–7.
[73] Kleindorfer D, Broderick J, Demaerschalk B, et al. Cost of alteplase has more than doubled over the past decade. Stroke 2017;48(7):2000–2.

[74] Gasior AC, Knott EM, Sharp SW, et al. Experience with an evidence-based protocol using fibrinolysis as first line treatment for empyema in children. J Pediatr Surg 2013;48(6):1312–5.
[75] Cohen E, Mahant S, Dell SD, et al. The long-term outcomes of pediatric pleural empyema: a prospective study. Arch Pediatr Adolesc Med 2012;166(11):999–1004.
[76] Redden MD, Chin TY, van Driel ML. Surgical versus non-surgical management for pleural empyema. Cochrane Database Syst Rev 2017;(3):CD010651.
[77] Livingston MH, Cohen E, Giglia L, et al. Are some children with empyema at risk for treatment failure with fibrinolytics? A multicenter cohort study. J Pediatr Surg 2016;51(5):832–7.
[78] Rahman NM, Maskell NA, West A, et al. Intrapleural use of tissue plasminogen activator and DNase in pleural infection. N Engl J Med 2011;365(6):518–26.
[79] Livingston MH, Mahant S, Ratjen F, et al. Intrapleural dornase and tissue plasminogen activator in pediatric empyema (DTPA): a study protocol for a randomized controlled trial. Trials 2017;18(1):293.
[80] Dotson K, Timm N, Gittelman M. Is spontaneous pneumothorax really a pediatric problem? A national perspective. Pediatr Emerg Care 2012;28(4):340–4.
[81] Guimaraes CV, Donnelly LF, Warner BW. CT findings for blebs and bullae in children with spontaneous pneumothorax and comparison with findings in normal age-matched controls. Pediatr Radiol 2007;37(9):879–84.
[82] Laituri CA, Valusek PA, Rivard DC, et al. The utility of computed tomography in the management of patients with spontaneous pneumothorax. J Pediatr Surg 2011;46(8):1523–5.
[83] Robinson PD, Cooper P, Ranganathan SC. Evidence-based management of paediatric primary spontaneous pneumothorax. Paediatr Respir Rev 2009;10(3):110–7.
[84] MacDuff A, Arnold A, Harvey J. on behalf of the BTS Pleural Disease Guideline Group. Management of spontaneous pneumothorax: British Thoracic Society pleural disease guideline 2010. Thorax 2010;65:ii18–31.
[85] Baumann MH, Strange C, Heffner JE, et al. Management of spontaneous pneumothorax. Chest 2001;119:590–602.
[86] Williams K, Baumann L, Grabowski J, et al. Current practice in the management of spontaneous pneumothorax in children. J Laparoendosc Adv Surg Tech A 2019;29(4):551–6.
[87] Cook CH, Melvin WS, Groner JI, et al. A cost-effective thoracoscopic treatment strategy for pediatric spontaneous pneumothorax. Surg Endosc 1999;13:1208–10.
[88] Williams K, Lautz TB, Leon AH, et al. Optimal timing of video-assisted thoracoscopic surgery for primary spontaneous pneumothorax in children. J Pediatr Surg 2018;53:1858–61.
[89] Young Choi S, Beom Park C, Wha Song S, et al. What factors predict recurrence after an initial episode of primary spontaneous pneumothorax in children? Ann Thorac Cardiovasc Surg 2014;20(6):961–7.
[90] Lopez ME, Fallon SC, Lee TC, et al. Management of the pediatric spontaneous pneumothorax: is primary surgery the treatment of choice? Am J Surg 2014;208:571–6.
[91] Soler LM, Raymond SL, Larson SD, et al. Initial primary spontaneous pneumothorax in children and adolescents: operate or wait? J Pediatr Surg 2018;53:1960–3.
[92] Qureshi FG, Sandulache VC, Richardson W, et al. Primary vs delayed surgery for spontaneous pneumothorax in children: which is better? J Pediatr Surg 2005;40:166–9.
[93] Butterworth SA, Blair GK, LeBlanc JG, et al. An open and shut case for early VATS treatment of primary spontaneous pneumothorax in children. Can J Surg 2007;50:171–4.
[94] Chambers A, Scarci M. In patients with first-episode primary spontaneous pneumothorax is video-assisted thoracoscopic surgery superior to tube thoracostomy alone in terms of time to resolution of pneumothorax and incidence of recurrence? Interact Cardiovasc Thorac Surg 2009;9:1003–8.
[95] Noppen M, Alexander P, Driesen P, et al. Manual aspiration versus chest tube drainage in first episodes of primary spontaneous pneumothorax: a multicenter, prospective, randomized pilot study. Am J Respir Crit Care Med 2002;165:1240–4.

[96] Williams K, Oyetunji TA, Hsuing G, et al. Spontaneous pneumothorax in children: national management strategies and outcomes. J Laparoendosc Adv Surg Tech A 2018;28:218–22.
[97] Leys CM, Hirschl RB, Kohler JE, et al. Changing the paradigm for management of pediatric primary spontaneous pneumothorax: a simple aspiration test predicts need for operation. J Pediatr Surg 2020;55(1):169–75.
[98] Bialas RC, Weiner TM, Phillips JD. Video-assisted thoracic surgery for primary spontaneous pneumothorax in children: is there an optimal technique? J Pediatr Surg 2008;43:2151–5.
[99] Sudduth CL, Shinnick JK, Geng Z, et al. Optimal surgical technique in spontaneous pneumothorax: a systematic review and meta-analysis. J Surg Res 2017;210:32–46.

Advances in Pediatrics 67 (2020) 171–182

ADVANCES IN PEDIATRICS

Overuse Injuries in Pediatric Athletes

Ryan Ridenour, MD[a], William Hennrikus, MD[b,*]

[a]Penn State College of Medicine; [b]Penn State College of Medicine, 30 Hope Drive, Hershey, PA 17033, USA

Keywords

• Overuse injury • Apophysitis • Pediatric • Athlete

Key points

- Overuse injuries in pediatric athletes are common.
- An understanding of tendon insertion anatomy is key.
- Most overuse injuries respond to conservative treatment strategies.

INTRODUCTION

Sports have become a pivotal aspect of American culture. With this increased interest among Americans, there has been an increase in sports participation in children and adolescents. According to the National Council of Youth Sports, nearly 60 million children participate in organized sports with approximately 50% of those participating in more than one sport [1]. In addition, children are playing sports year-round more so than in previous decades [1]. This increased participation has resulted in an increase in sports injuries.

With the advent of year-round training and multiple weekend games, many children and adolescents are not getting adequate rest [2]. The more intense training combined with the lack of rest places young athletes at heightened risk for overuse injuries of the upper extremity, lower extremity, and hip/pelvis. This evolution to increased focus on one sport and sport-specific work-out programs likely contributes to more overuse injuries [2].

Overuse injuries are related to repetitive stress applied to the musculoskeletal system without adequate time provided for recovery following the stress [1].

*Corresponding author. *E-mail address:* whennrikus@hmc.psu.edu

https://doi.org/10.1016/j.yapd.2020.04.001

Children are at an increased risk for overuse injury due to their immature skeletal system. Specifically, areas such as physeal-epiphyseal junctions, apophyses, or tendon-bone junctions are areas unique to children and sites where stress can lead to overuse injuries [1]. Prior epidemiologic studies examined the effect age and gender have on overuse injuries in adolescent high school students [1,3]. Overall, injury distribution was similar across all high school years [1,3]; however, girls tended to sustain injuries earlier in high school years compared with boys [1,3]. This finding may be related to the earlier skeletal maturity of girls compared with boys. Once the growth plates fuse, growth plate injuries decrease thereafter.

The purpose of this review was to provide a summary of common pediatric overuse injuries seen in sports. This article reviews Little League shoulder (LLS), Little League elbow, gymnast wrist, Osgood-Schlatter (OS) apophysitis, Sever apophysitis, Iselin apophysitis, and pelvic overuse injuries.

PEDIATRIC UPPER EXTREMITY OVERUSE INJURIES

Little league shoulder

LLS refers to an overuse injury to the proximal humeral physis. LLS is most often seen in patients between the ages of 11 and 16 years [1,4]. This particular overuse injury often stems from throwing a baseball. During the late cocking phase of throwing, the shoulder is placed into a maximum external rotation position and a maximal amount of torque is placed on the shoulder [4,5]. The late cocking position, in the young athlete, places stress across the proximal humeral physis that can lead to inflammation, microfracture, and physeal widening [1]. Youth athletes will complain of both pain and reduced velocity with pitching [1]. Physical examination demonstrates pain with palpation at the proximal anterolateral aspect of the humerus and associated pain with resisted shoulder motions [2]. Radiograph findings include widening at the physis, fragmentation, and sclerosis [2] (Fig. 1). Treatment of LLS involves rest, activity modification, nonsteroidal anti-inflammatory drugs (NSAIDs), and, in some cases, complete abstinence from throwing for 3 months. Subsequently, a progressive therapy protocol geared toward proper shoulder mechanics and throwing is implemented to allow a gradual return to play [4]. In most cases, these treatments lead to resolution; however, there are instances in which growth arrest and subsequent angular deformity can occur in severe cases. There are no long-term sequelae.

Little league elbow

Little League elbow encompasses a wide spectrum of disorders that includes fractures, apophysitis, avulsions, and delays in ossification [2]. The terminology "Little League elbow" is a common reference regarding multiple disorders causing pain around the elbow, many of which are not related to throwing a baseball. Most adolescent elbow injuries occur at the medial elbow and result from sports that place increased stress at the medial elbow. Although termed Little League elbow, sports that place stress at the medial elbow include

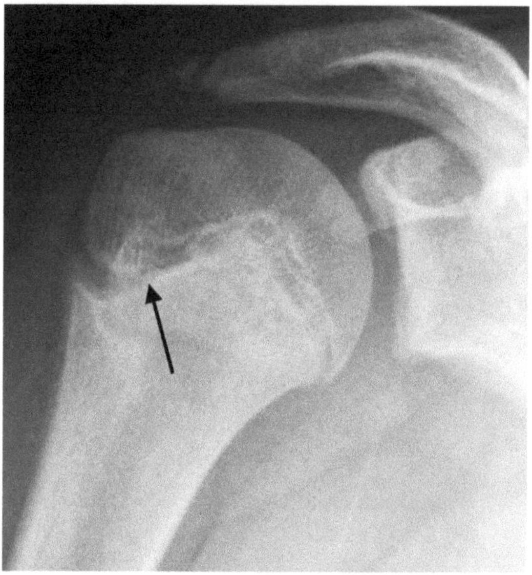

Fig. 1. LLS. In young pitchers, phases of throwing seen with baseball place stress across the proximal humerus physis that can lead to an overuse injury of the proximal humerus physis. This arrow notes sclerosis and changes at the proximal humerus physis consistent with LLS.

baseball, tennis, and gymnastics [6]. Physical examination demonstrates pain over the medial structures of the elbow, such as the medial epicondyle, flexor-pronator muscle origin, and ulnar collateral ligament. Reproduction of valgus stress to the elbow will reproduce pain. Radiographs are normal early on; however, with time radiographs may show widening at the apophysis or fragmentation [1]. Chronic repetitive stress in skeletally immature children can lead to avulsion injury at the medial epicondyle apophysis (Fig. 2). Skeletally mature high school athletes with repetitive stress can develop injury to the ulnar collateral ligament (UCL) rather than at the fused medial epicondyle [6] (Fig. 3). Specific motions at the elbow during the late cocking and acceleration phases of throwing, such as valgus and distraction, can lead to apophysitis and apophyseal avulsion injuries [2]. The medial epicondyle, UCL, and flexor-pronator origin receive high amounts of stress with throwing a baseball [1]. The mainstays of treatment include rest and activity modification [6]. In addition, a course of NSAIDs can help with pain [6]. Most athletes will need to take a rest from throwing for 6 weeks. If the symptoms do not resolve after 6 weeks of rest, advanced imaging in the form of MRI may be useful to determine the possible need for surgery [1]. The mainstay of treatment as described previously will typically lead to resolution of symptoms without long-term injury. In some cases of Little League elbow, long-term sequalae can include elbow instability, decreased range of motion, and pain.

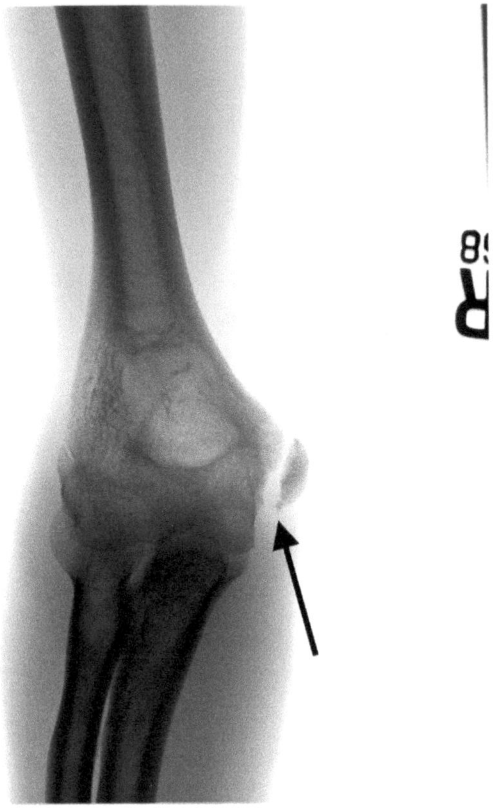

Fig. 2. Medial epicondyle avulsion. Little League elbow refers to injuries about the medial elbow. Often times, the medial collateral ligament will tear or avulse at the medial epicondyle leading to fracture in some instances. This arrow notes an avulsion at the medial epicondyle.

Gymnast wrist

Gymnast wrist refers to an overuse injury of the distal radial epiphysis. Gymnast wrist occurs in young athletes who repetitively bear weight on their upper extremities [1]. This disorder is most often seen in gymnastic athletes between the ages of 10 and 14 years [7,8]. Previous studies have reported that more than 50% of competitive youth gymnasts complain of wrist pain [8]. The balance beam, floor exercises, and pommel horse were the events most associated with wrist pain [8]. Because the radius absorbs more load compared with the ulna, gymnast wrist results in radial epiphysitis more often than ulnar epiphysitis. The injury stems from both compression and hyperextension forces on the physis [7]. Physical examination demonstrates tenderness to palpation at the distal radial physis. Occasionally tenderness can arise at the ulnar physis as well. Initial radiographs may be normal. In time, the radiographs show

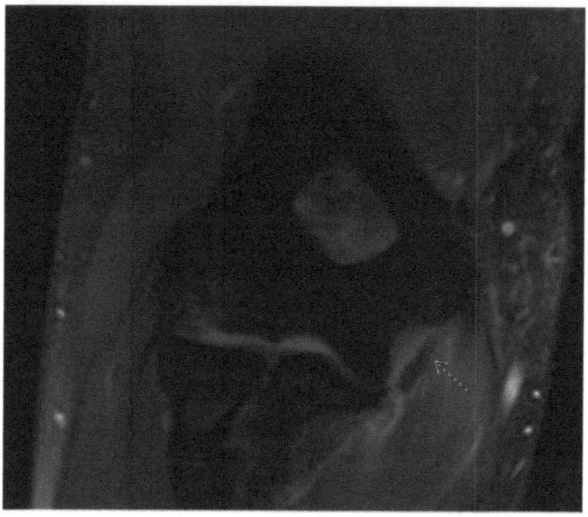

Fig. 3. UCL tear. As children mature, the physis closes. As the physis closes, stress applied to specific joints changes from stress on the physis to stress on the ligament. In some instances, this can lead to a UCL tear. This arrow notes a tear of the UCL at the medial elbow in a mature high school athlete.

widening and sclerosis at the distal radial physis [7] (Fig. 4). Treatment includes rest, a wrist brace, and NSAIDs [7]. If conservative treatment fails, advanced imaging in the form of MRI can be used to assess for growth arrest, soft tissue tears, and the possible need for surgery. Long-term sequelae from gymnast wrist is not uncommon. Chronic pain and decreased motion can occur.

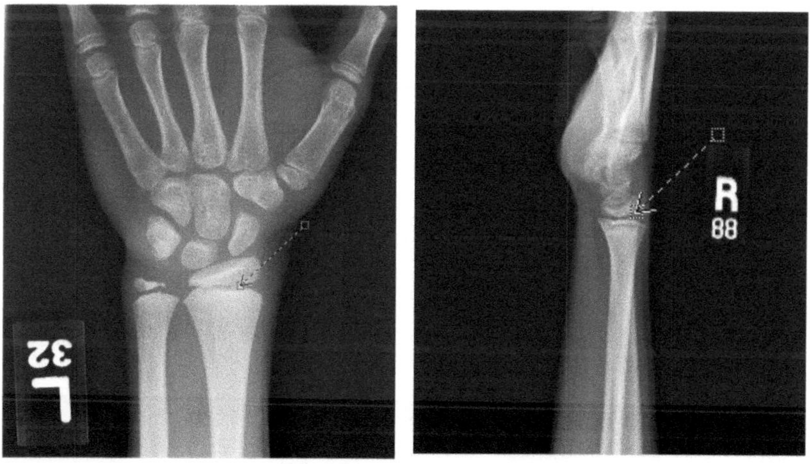

Fig. 4. Gymnast wrist. Gymnast wrist refers to a hyperextension injury seen in children at the distal radius epiphysis. Repetitive stress and hyperextension moments create an area of tension and weakness at the physis. This arrow notes sclerotic changes at the distal radius physis in a patient with gymnast wrist.

PEDIATRIC LOWER EXTREMITY OVERUSE INJURIES

Osgood-Schlatter apophysitis

OS apophysitis is one of the most common knee disorders seen in the young athlete. OS is caused by a traction injury at the patellar tendon insertion on the tibia at the tibial tubercle. Repetitive traction at this area can lead to inflammation, microfracture, and calcification of the tibial tubercle apophysis [9]. It is common to see OS in young athletes (10–15 years old) who are active in sports related to running, jumping, and pivoting, such as soccer or basketball [1,9]. OS is a clinical diagnosis. Most patients will present with pain at the tibial tubercle. Palpation of the tibial tubercle will elicit tenderness. Radiographs confirm the clinical diagnosis and can be useful to rule out red flag diagnoses, such as fracture, infection, or bone tumor [9]. Radiographs in patients who have chronic OS demonstrate swelling, fragmentation of apophysis, and calcifications within the patellar tendon [2,9] (Fig. 5). OS is usually a self-limited disorder. Treatment includes NSAIDs, brief periods of rest, ice, and activity modifications. Children can continue to participate in their sport as long as pain improves with conservative care. A knee strap or pad over the knee may help to prevent trauma or relieve direct pressure over the tubercle [1,9]. In more severe cases, a course of physical therapy, a 1-month period of rest from sports, and/or a 1-month period of knee immobilization in a brace may be indicated [9]. OS does not have a quick fix, and most youth athletes will benefit from a treatment strategy of repeat prescriptions of conservative care for repeat episodes of pain.

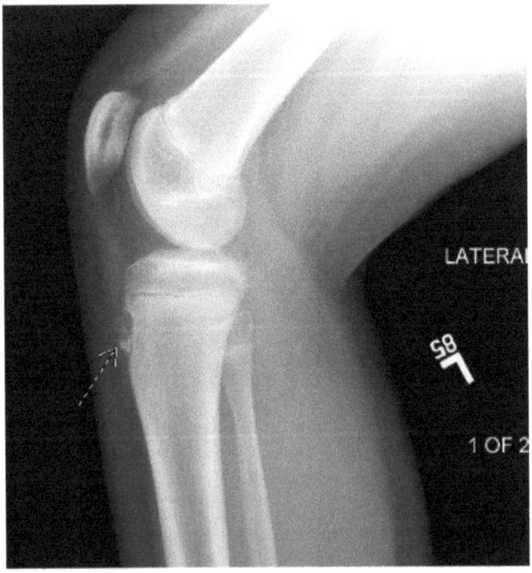

Fig. 5. OS disease. OS disease refers to a disorder at the tibial tubercle that arises from repetitive stress from the patellar tendon's insertion at the tubercle. This arrow notes fragmentation and changes at the tubercle related to OS disease.

Symptoms completely resolve once the athlete reaches skeletal maturity, typically age 14 years in girls and 16 years in boys [2]. Long-term complications are rare [2]; however, surgery may be indicated in rare cases of a persistent painful bump after skeletal maturity [10].

Sever apophysitis

Sever apophysitis most often affects children ages 8 to 13 years who participate in cleated sports, such as soccer and football, or high-impact sports, such as gymnastics or basketball [1]. Sever apophysitis presents with heal pain localized to the calcaneal apophysis in the growing child. Overuse stress at this site is caused by the pull of the Achilles tendon, the plantar fascia, and direct impact to the heel. The pediatric athlete will often describe pain from the medial to the lateral aspect of the posterior calcaneus [1,2]. Risk factors for this disorder include obesity, wearing poorly padded cleats, and high-impact physical activity [11]. The diagnosis often can be made based on clinic examination. The athlete will demonstrate tenderness along the posterior calcaneus.

Radiographs confirm the clinical diagnosis and can be useful to rule out more serious diagnoses, such as a bone cyst or stress fracture. Radiographs can be read as normal and typically demonstrate sclerosis and fragmentation at the calcaneus apophysis [11] (Fig. 6). Treatment includes rest, ice, Achilles stretching exercises, placing a gel pad in the cleats, using sneakers rather than cleats for practice, and NSAIDs. In severe cases, a 4-week course of immobilization with a controlled ankle motion (CAM) boot may be indicated. As symptoms improve, children may begin to gradually return to sports [1,2]. If symptoms worsen, MRI may be considered to rule out a possible calcaneus stress fracture [1]. In general, similar to OS disease, Sever apophysitis can have a waxing and waning course until skeletal maturity. Rather than suggesting that treatment is curative, a management strategy including repeat prescriptions of conservative care until skeletal maturity is often needed. After closure

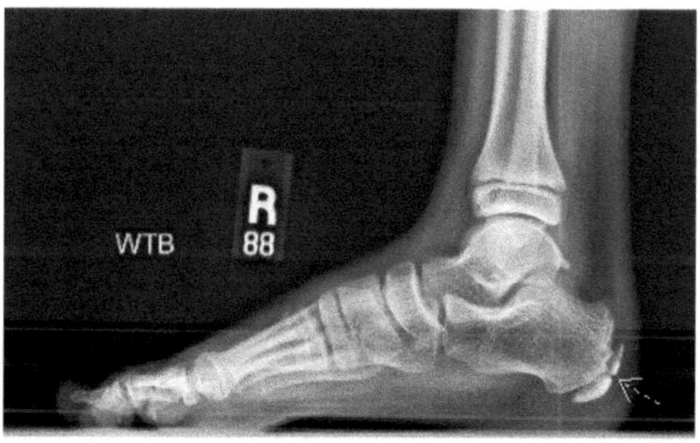

Fig. 6. Sever apophysitis. Sever apophysitis involves a chronic overuse injury at the posterior calcaneus. This arrow notes changes related to chronic apophysitis at the posterior calcaneus.

of the growth plates, there is usually no long-term lasting detriment to the child. There are no long-term sequalae following Sever apophysitis.

Iselin apophysitis

Iselin apophysitis is an overuse injury related to traction on the apophysis at the base of the fifth metatarsal at the site of the peroneal brevis insertion [12]. Repetitive stress of running and jumping leads to pain and inflammation at this apophysis [13]. Chronic stress leads to ossification and a small bump at the base of the fifth metatarsal [13]. Iselin apophysitis most often occurs in adolescents [12]. Athletes complain of lateral foot pain and a small bump. Physical examination demonstrates swelling, tenderness, and a protuberance at the base of the fifth metatarsal at the peroneal brevis insertion [13]. Resisted ankle eversion will cause pain at this apophysis. Radiographs are helpful to rule out a fifth metatarsal avulsion fracture or stress fracture. Radiographs demonstrate sclerosis and fragmentation parallel to the fifth metatarsal (Fig. 7). A stress fracture or an avulsion fracture occurs perpendicular to the fifth metatarsal. Treatment includes rest, ice, and NSAIDs to help with pain [13]. Often, a 4-week course of immobilization in a CAM boot is indicated [13]. Last, as with OS apophysitis and Sever apophysitis, a waxing and waning course of symptomatology is common. Recommending a management strategy including repeat prescriptions of conservative care until skeletal maturity is often needed.

PEDIATRIC HIP AND PELVIS OVERUSE INJURIES

There are numerous areas around the hip and pelvis that are sources for overuse injuries in the growing athlete. Specifically, 6 major sites of large tendon attachments exist in the pediatric hip and pelvis. These sites are common areas for apophysitis and avulsion fractures because of the soft cartilaginous nature of the apophysis and the strong pull of tendons [1]. These 6 sites include the

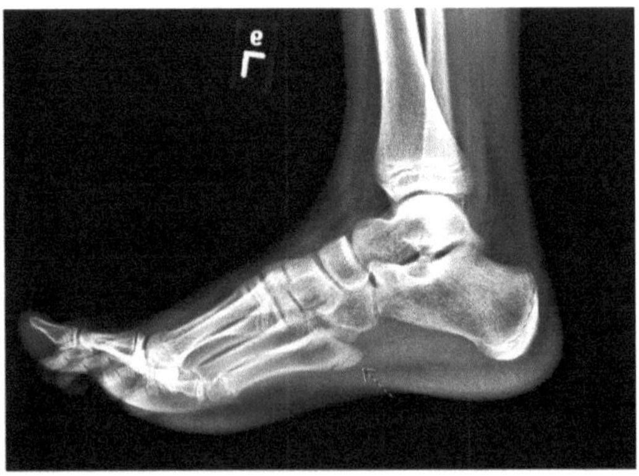

Fig. 7. Iselin apophysitis. Iselin apophysitis refers to a traction injury to the apophysis of the fifth metatarsal base. This radiograph demonstrates the sequelae of Iselin disease with fragmentation at the base of the fifth metatarsal.

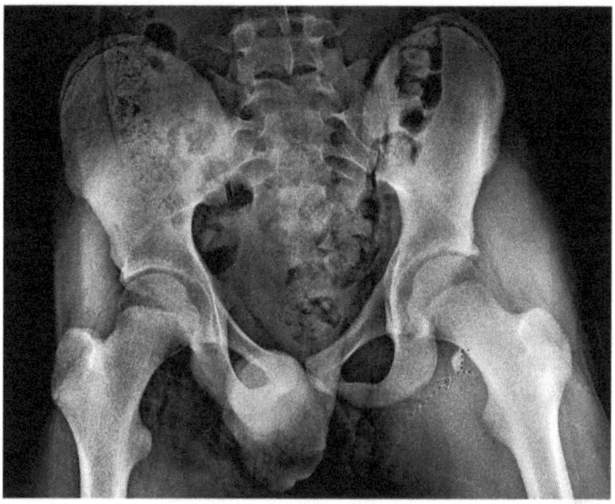

Fig. 8. Disorders of the hip and pelvis. There are 6 different overuse injuries that can result in avulsions of tendon insertion sites of the hip or pelvis. This arrow notes an avulsion at the lesser trochanter stemming from the pull of the iliopsoas tendon.

anterior superior iliac spine (ASIS), Sartorius tendon origin; the iliac crest, tensor fascia tendon origin and abdominal muscles insertion; the anterior inferior iliac spine (AIIS), rectus femoris tendon origin; the ischial tuberosity, hamstring origin: the greater trochanter, gluteus maximus insertion and external hip rotator muscle insertion; and the lesser trochanter, iliopsoas tendon insertion [1]. A force strong enough to cause a ligamentous or tendon tear in adults will cause an apophyseal avulsion injury in the child athlete due to the soft and weak nature of the apophysis at these locations [14]. Complete separation of the apophysis from an acute tendon pull, as well as chronic

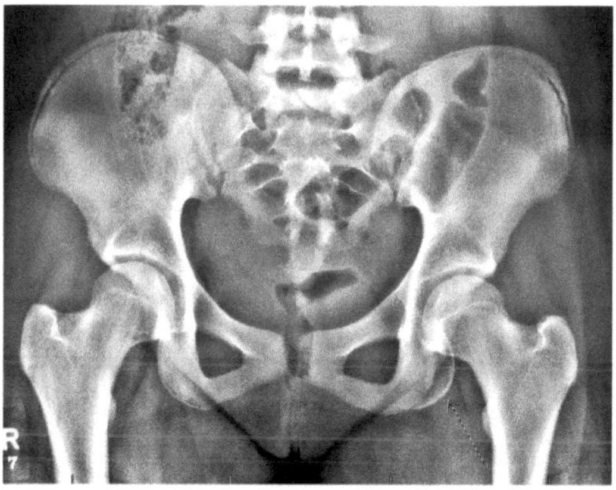

Fig. 9. Disorders of the hip and pelvis. This arrow notes an avulsion at the ischial tuberosity stemming from the pull of the hamstring tendons.

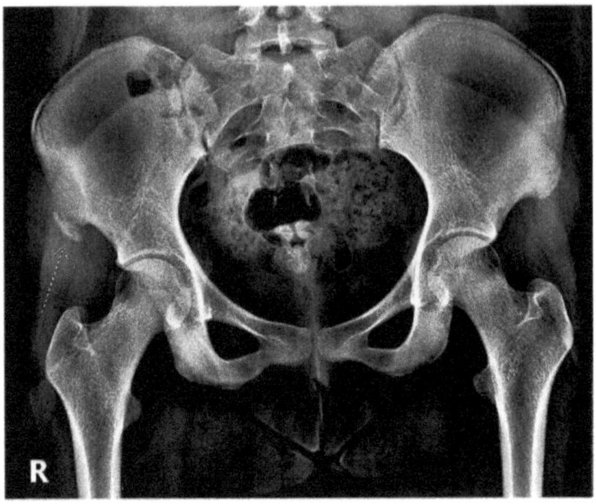

Fig. 10. Disorders of the hip and pelvis. This arrow notes an avulsion at the ASIS stemming from the pull of the Sartorius tendon.

traction injuries leading to apophysitis can occur [14]. The pediatric athlete presents with pain and a limp about the hip or pelvis in the region of the injured apophysis. Physical examination demonstrates pain with palpation over the apophysis and pain with resisted provocative muscle contracture. An anteroposterior pelvis radiograph is indicated when suspicion for a hip or pelvic apophyseal injury occurs (Figs. 8–12). The radiograph may show a displaced avulsion of the injured apophysis. Treatment of hip and pelvic apophyseal avulsion injuries includes rest from sports, partial weight bearing with crutches, ice, and NSAIDs [1] In most cases, weight bearing can be returned to normal at 4 weeks and a return to gradual sports can occur at approximately 8 weeks.

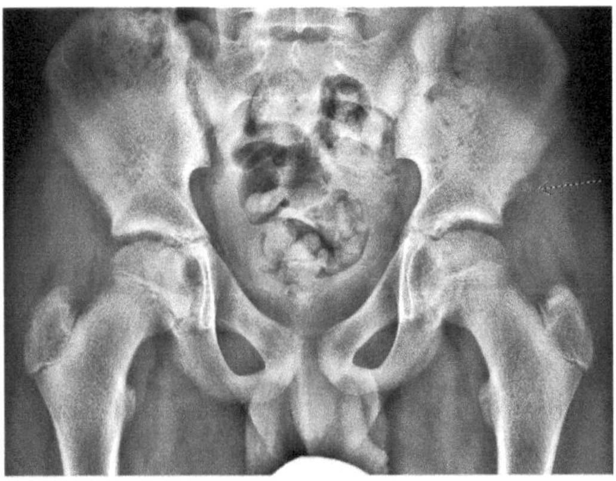

Fig. 11. Disorders of the hip and pelvis. This arrow notes an avulsion at the AIIS stemming from the pull of the rectus femoris tendon.

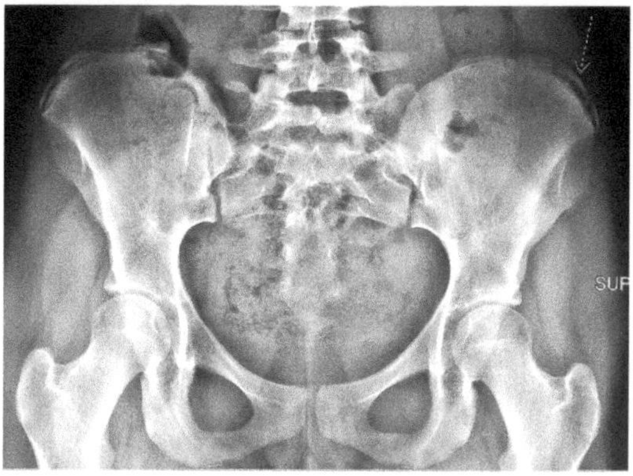

Fig. 12. Disorders of the hip and pelvis. This arrow notes an avulsion at the iliac crest stemming from the pull of the tensor fascia tendon.

Some investigators suggest operative treatment if the apophysis is displaced >2 cm [15]. Most cases heal on their own with conservative measures. Those children who do require surgery, most often go on to union of the avulsed fragment. There are not usually long-term effects on function following these injuries.

SUMMARY

Overuse injuries in pediatric and adolescent athletes are on the rise. Children are participating in competitive sports at a younger age and are focusing on participating in a single sport on a year-round basis. Educating parents and coaches about the dangers of year-round single-sport training in young athletes is paramount to help prevent these injuries. In addition, once an overuse injury occurs, recognizing the signs and symptoms, understanding the basic musculoskeletal anatomy including tendon insertion sites, and obtaining imaging studies are key to making the diagnosis. Early diagnosis and appropriate treatment helps return the athlete to play in a timely fashion and prevents long-term sequelae.

Disclosure

The authors have no disclosures.

References

[1] Magrini D, Dahab K. Musculoskeletal overuse injuries in the pediatric population. Curr Sports Med Rep 2016;15(6):392–9.
[2] Wu M, Fallon R, Heyworth B. Overuse injuries in the pediatric population. Sports Med Arthrosc Rev 2016;24(4):150–8.
[3] Schroeder A, Comstock R, Collins C, et al. Epidemiology of overuse injuries among high school athletes in the United States. J Pediatr 2015;166(3):600–6.
[4] Osbahr D, Kim H, Dugas J. Little league shoulder. Curr Opin Pediatr 2010;22(1):35–40.

[5] Pappas A, Zawacki R, Sullivan T. Biomechanics of baseball pitching. A preliminary report. Am J Sports Med 1985;13(4):216–22.
[6] Leahy I, Schorpion M, Ganley T. Common medial elbow injuries in the adolescent athlete. J Hand Ther 2015;28:201–11.
[7] Ellington M, Edmonds E. Pediatric elbow and wrist pathology related to sports participation. Orthop Clin North Am 2016;47:743–8.
[8] DiFiori J, Puffer J, Aish B, et al. Wrist pain in young gymnasts: frequency and effects upon training over 1 year. Clin J Sports Med 2002;12(6):348–53.
[9] Smith J, Varacallo M. Osgood Schlatter's disease (tibial tubercle apophysitis). Treasure Island (FL): StatPearls; 2019.
[10] Weiss JM, Jordan SS, Anderson JS, et al. Surgical treatment of unresolved Osgood Schlatter disease: ossicle resection with tibial tubercleplasty. J Pediatr Orthop 2007;27:844–7.
[11] Ramponi D, Baker C. Sever's disease (calcaneal apophysitis). Adv Emerg Nurs J 2019;41(1):10–4.
[12] Sylvester JE, Hennrikus WL. Treatment outcomes of adolescents with Iselin's apophysitis. J Pediatr Orthop 2015;24:362–5.
[13] Forrester R, Eyre-Brook A, Mannan K. Iselin's disease: a systematic review. J Foot Ankle Surg 2017;56:1065–9.
[14] Young S, Safran MR. Greater trochanter apophysitis in the adolescent athlete. Clin J Sports Med 2015;25:57–8.
[15] Arner JW, McClincy MP, Bradley JP. Hamstring injuries in athletes: evidence based treatment. J Am Acad Orthop Surg 2019;27:868–77.

Advances in Pediatrics 67 (2020) 183–196

ADVANCES IN PEDIATRICS

New Developments in Diagnosis, Treatment, and Management of Duchenne Muscular Dystrophy

Maria Gieron-Korthals, MD[a,*], Raymond Fernandez, MD[b,c]

[a]Department of Pediatrics, Division of Child Neurology, University of South Florida, Morsani College of Medicine, 17 Davis Boulevard, Suite 200, Tampa, FL 33606, USA; [b]Pediatric Neurology Associates, 4150 North Armenia Avenue, Suite 103, Tampa, FL 33607, USA; [c]Muscular Dystrophy Association Care Center, Shriners Hospital for Children, Tampa, FL, USA

Keywords

• Duchenne • Dystrophin gene and protein • Exon skipping • Gene transfer

Key points

- Duchenne muscular dystrophy (DMD) is an X-linked, recessive, lethal disease characterized by progressive loss of muscle strength and function. Becker muscular dystrophy is less severe, although there is phenotypic overlap with DMD.
- Mutations in the dystrophin gene cause absence of or an insufficiently functional dystrophin protein that destabilizes the muscle fiber membrane.
- Respiratory, cardiac, orthopedic, and other comorbidities contribute to disability and shorten life span.
- The clinical course and survival time of patients with DMD are changing because of advances in diagnostic testing, management of comorbidities, and evolving molecular and genetic treatments, such as exon skipping and gene transfer, in addition to corticosteroids.
- Neonatal screening is feasible but not yet being performed. Earlier diagnosis will become more critical as treatments improve.

HISTORICAL REVIEW

The dystrophin gene was cloned in 1987 [1]. The dystrophin gene was found to be on the X chromosome at the Xp21 site based on a cytogenetic study of

*Corresponding author. *E-mail address:* mgieron@usf.edu

https://doi.org/10.1016/j.yapd.2020.03.002
0065-3101/20/

girls with the Duchenne muscular dystrophy (DMD) phenotype and X-autosome translocation [2], by linkage analysis [3] and by a cytogenetic study of a boy with DMD and 3 additional mutations, all within a large deletion in the Xp21 band [4]. The identification of the gene product, dystrophin, was accomplished in 1987 [5]. Subsequent work focused on refining techniques for precise genetic diagnosis and more detailed information on dystrophin.

It is important to realize that before the availability of DMD gene analysis, the diagnosis of DMD/Becker muscular dystrophy (BMD) was based on history (including family history), physical examination, serum creatine kinase (CK) level, and muscle biopsy histopathology, all of which may not result in a specific diagnosis. It was sometimes learned later that the reasonably established diagnosis of DMD/BMD was not correct because there is phenotypic mimicry caused by mutations in other genes. However, diagnostic errors are now uncommon.

DYSTROPHIN, THE DUCHENNE MUSCULAR DYSTROPHY GENE PRODUCT

Dystrophin is an intracellular muscle fiber protein in close proximity to the inner surface of the muscle fiber membrane. Its primary function is to stabilize the membrane during muscle contraction. This stabilization is accomplished by a series of direct connections to other intracellular and transmembrane proteins and then by indirect extension to extracellular proteins that provide basement membrane integrity.

There are 4 functional units of the dystrophin gene (Fig. 1):

1. The N terminus or actin-binding domain, which binds with the muscle contractile protein, actin [6].
2. The central rod domain made up of 24 spectrinlike repeat units with 4 interspersed hinge units that provide flexibility during muscle contraction [7].
3. The cysteine-rich domain, which connects dystrophin to the transmembrane protein, beta-dystroglycan, which in turn connects to other transmembrane proteins, including sarcospan and the tightly knit sarcoglycan proteins within the muscle fiber membrane. Beta-dystroglycan connects to alpha-dystroglycan via its extracellular extension providing a link to laminin-2, a significant component of the extracellular basement membrane [8].
4. The carboxy-terminus, which connects dystrophin with the intracellular proteins, dystrobrexin and syntrophins, that function in neuromuscular synaptic maintenance and also function to stabilize neuronal nitric oxide synthase (nNOS) to the muscle fiber membrane. nNOS is an enzyme that catalyzes nitric oxide formation, a signaling molecule that modulates vascular tone. If nNOS is not attached to the muscle fiber membrane because of lack of dystrophin, functional ischemia occurs as the result of blood vessel constriction.

The pathology of dystrophin deficiency is multifaceted. Primarily, the integrity of the muscle fiber membrane is compromised because of breakdown during muscle fiber contraction allowing leakage of toxic substances into muscle fibers, notably calcium. Another factor is the loss of membrane nNOS, causing

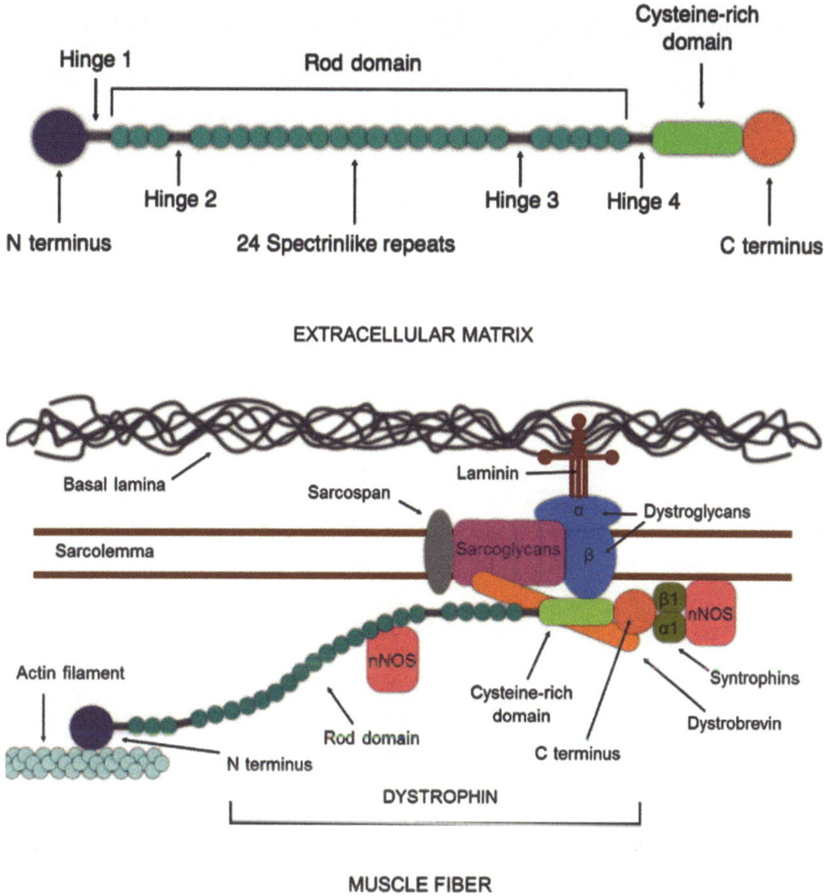

Fig. 1. Dystrophin and the dystrophin-associated glycoprotein complex (DAGC). (*Top*) Dystrophin protein. The N-terminal and C-terminal regions contain functionally important binding sites, whereas the rod domain acts as a linker. (*Bottom*) Dystrophin connects the cytoskeleton to the sarcolemma via components of the DAGC, a large multiprotein complex that includes laminin, sarcoglycans, α-dystroglycan and β-dystroglycan, sarcospan, dystrobrevin, and α1-syntrophin and β1-syntrophin, as well as associated proteins such as nitric oxide synthase. nNOS, neuronal nitric oxide synthase. (*From* Douglas AG, Wood MJ. *Splicing therapy for neuromuscular disease.* Mol Cell Neurosci. 2013; 56: 169–185; with permission.)

vasoconstriction and muscle ischemia and muscle fiber necrosis. This loss causes inflammation, resulting in further damage and replacement of muscle fibers by fat and fibrous tissue. Increase in oxidative stress and recruitment of muscle fiber satellite cells are also implicated in dystrophin deficiency [9–13].

CLINICAL MANIFESTATIONS OF DUCHENNE MUSCULAR DYSTROPHY

DMD affects 1 in approximately 3600 to 6000 male births. The pathology of the disease, progressive muscle fiber breakdown at an accelerated pace, begins in utero, as shown by serum CK level increases detectable at birth [14]. However, there is a delayed onset of clinical symptoms and signs that typically begins early, although it is not always distinct. Without a high level of suspicion, the diagnosis of DMD is often not established until about 4 to 5 years of age. Although motor delay and weakness are the hallmarks of DMD, many boys show early cognitive and behavioral abnormalities that are sometimes more obvious and of more significance. This finding should not shift attention away from the possibility of underlying muscle disease; it should reinforce the likelihood of DMD because many boys simultaneously show early speech, language, and cognitive delays as well as behaviors suggestive of autism spectrum disorder [15]. A simple and sensitive but nonspecific serum CK measurement serves as a reliable screen for DMD because it is always increased.

With a focus mainly on motor development, early differences in young boys with DMD compared with typically developing peers are common [16]. Note that these differences are not always thought to be significant, because young boys with DMD usually show functional motor improvement that can continue to 5 to 6 years of age, at which time they plateau and typically begin to decline by age 7 years.

The more obvious signs of muscle weakness that are abnormal at any age include the Gower maneuver when shifting position against gravity; difficulty climbing stairs; waddling gait, indicating hip girdle weakness; and bulky muscle groups, especially calves (pseudohypertrophy). These signs should lead to the measurement of serum CK level. Nonspecific clumsiness and toe walking in the absence of muscle weakness should also prompt serum CK measurement.

A common scenario is detection of increased serum transaminases, alanine transaminase (ALT) and aspartate transaminase (AST) levels, when a comprehensive metabolic panel is ordered for a variety of reasons, often not because of suspected muscle disease. This finding often triggers a referral to a gastroenterologist because of the increase in liver enzyme levels. However, in the absence of clinically evident liver disease, the finding of increased transaminase levels should be followed by serum CK measurement, which is not on the routine comprehensive metabolic panel. The CK level will be increased to a significantly higher degree than ALT and AST, leading to muscle disease as the source. This finding saves time and unnecessary testing, which is sometimes invasive and expensive.

Boys with DMD can experience improvement in motor function until the age of approximately 4 to 6 years. Following this, they enter the plateau stage of their disease, which can be as short as a few months to possibly 1 year, at which time they invariably decline relentlessly. Identification of these stages is important because it guides management, which becomes more complex as the disease advances.

Female carriers may have varying degrees of muscle pain or weakness. Symptoms occur in up to 10% of female carriers and become more frequent with advancing age. Rarely, girls experience symptoms during childhood.

Even less common are girls with the severe DMD phenotype, as is seen in boys [17]. The presence or absence of symptoms are both determined by random inactivation of an X chromosome, which occurs early in embryogenesis. Carriers are at risk of developing cardiomyopathy, although the natural history has not been well characterized. Occult abnormalities can be found by echocardiogram and by cardiovascular MRI. Cardiac assessment of asymptomatic carriers is recommended every 3 to 5 years, beginning in young adulthood, or more often if symptomatic [18].

CARRIER DETECTION

Approximately two-thirds of mothers of boys with DMD are carriers. Carrier testing can be targeted in mothers and other at-risk women in the family, looking for the mutation in the proband. If a woman is a somatic cell line carrier, recurrence risk in future pregnancies is 50% for the disease in boys and 50% for girls to be carriers [19]. If a woman is not a somatic cell line carrier, the recurrence risk is low, but not zero. Parents must understand that recurrence is a possibility because of germ cell line mosaicism, with risk as high as 15%. Germ cell line mosaicism means that the mutation is present in some of the eggs in the woman's ovaries, and this cannot be detected by genetic testing before fertilization. This situation should be carefully explained so that parents can pursue all options regarding family planning and prevention of DMD in future pregnancies, both the disease and carrier state.

Carrier detection should be offered to all adult women within a family who are potential carriers. Children should be tested only if there is a medically compelling reason to do so, such as childhood onset of symptoms suspicious of muscle disease or cardiomyopathy.

Asymptomatic children who are potential carriers should not be tested. However, testing should be offered promptly when they reach the age of consent and are capable of making their own decisions regarding reproductive issues. Parents might request carrier detection in their young children because they are concerned about the possibility and simply want to know. This reason is not compelling, and clinicians are not obligated to comply.

Referral to a genetic counselor is recommended for advice, given the complexity of the issues involved.

GENETIC TESTING

Approximately 70% of DMD mutations are single-exon or multiexon deletions or duplications. The remainder are subexonic, including small deletions (as small as a single nucleotide), small insertions, nonsense mutations, and missense mutations, which are rarely pathogenic [20].

The diagnosis of DMD should be established by genetic testing, which has become more readily available and usually affordable with reasonable turnaround time. If affordability is an issue, funding sources are usually available and easily accessed in the multispecialty care center (MCC) setting.

The preferred initial testing method is next-generation sequencing (NGS) using a single-step method of data collection [21,22]. This method is generally being used in place of earlier 2-step methods involving multiplex ligation-dependent probe amplification or whole-genome microarray to look for exon-level deletions or duplications and, if necessary, followed by Sanger sequencing analysis to look for sequence abnormalities. If a mutation is detected by NGS and the data are convincing based on stringent criteria, confirmation by another method is not necessary.

If the clinical suspicion of DMD is high, targeted DMD gene analysis should be performed as the initial test. If targeted DMD gene analysis is negative, an appropriately expanded multigene panel should then be analyzed [23].

In contrast, if there is a reasonable degree of uncertainty regarding the diagnosis of DMD, an expanded gene panel that includes the DMD gene should be the initial diagnostic step [24]. Rarely, in less than 1% of boys with DMD, the genetic abnormality cannot be detected and a muscle biopsy is necessary. The biopsy specimen should be processed by a well-equipped laboratory and interpreted by an experienced muscle pathologist.

The algorithm for genetic testing is outlined in Fig. 2.

NEWBORN SCREENING FOR DUCHENNE MUSCULAR DYSTROPHY

DMD newborn screening is not yet being performed but is possible by measurement of CK level on a dried blood spot obtained shortly after birth. If the CK level is greater than 2000 IU/L, genetic testing is necessary [14]. If less than 2000 IU/L, CK measurement should be repeated in several weeks.

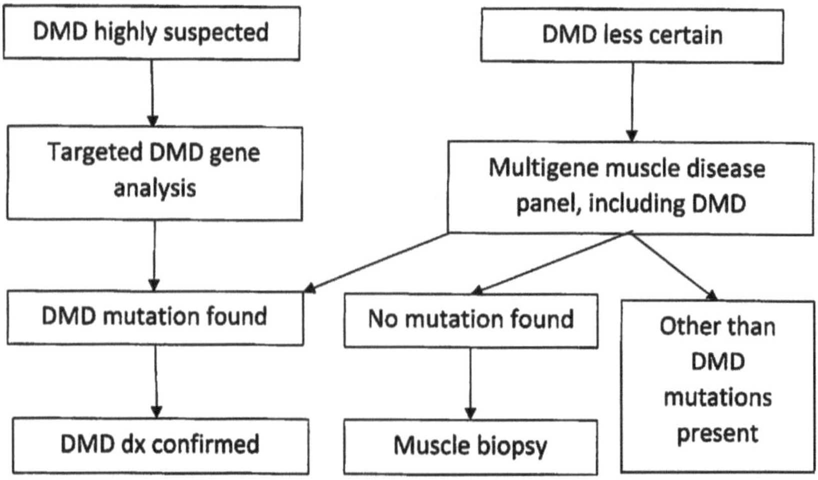

Fig. 2. A proposed algorithm for genetic testing for highly and less highly suspected DMD. dx, diagnosis.

GENOTYPE-PHENOTYPE CORRELATION

Most mutations that cause DMD are deletions that shift the translational reading frame of messenger RNA (mRNA), referred to as frameshift or out-of-frame deletions. In-frame deletions typically cause the milder BMD phenotype. Phenotypic expression largely depends on whether or not the mRNA reading frame is shifted at the deletion site [25].

A frameshift occurs when the number of nucleotides deleted is not a multiple of 3 [20]. Codons are nucleotide triplets that encode an amino acid during RNA translation in ribosomes. If the number of nucleotides deleted is not a multiple of 3, codons that are upstream from the mutation site encode normal amino acids up to the mutation site. However, codons downstream from the mutation site are out of frame and encode amino acids that are foreign to the remaining portion of the dystrophin protein. The result is the formation of unstable or virtually absent dystrophin, which causes the DMD phenotype.

In-frame deletions occur when the number of nucleotides deleted is a multiple of 3. Codons that are both upstream and downstream from the mutation site encode amino acids that are typically present and in proper sequence except for those deleted. This condition results in the formation of an internally truncated dystrophin protein that is semifunctional, causing the milder BMD phenotype.

There is an approximately 90% correlation between a frameshift deletion and the DMD phenotype [26]. However, there are exceptions to the reading frame rule to be considered when discussing possible clinical severity in young children. In-frame mutations predicting a milder phenotype are less certain. Also, it is difficult, if not impossible, to predict clinical severity caused by duplications [20].

Notable exceptions to the reading frame rule occur in boys with mutations before exon 6. This condition is caused by alternate translation initiation sites within ribosomes that become activated [27]. Reliable predictions within this region of the gene are difficult and families should be counseled accordingly. Another exception to the reading frame rule are boys that have frameshift deletions that are amenable to exon 44 skipping, often causing a milder DMD phenotype that resembles BMD [28]. This condition is probably caused by spontaneous skipping of exon 44, which restores the mutation to being in frame.

Boys with nonsense mutations that cause the formation of a premature stop codon typically show the DMD phenotype. Nonsense mutations result in an aberrantly located stop codon that stops dystrophin production prematurely, which triggers a process referred to as nonsense-mediated decay, and dystrophin is virtually absent. Although the DMD phenotype is often predicted accurately, there are exceptions, and a milder DMD phenotype may result. This condition is caused by spontaneous skipping of the exon that contains the premature stop codon, enabling the production of partially functional dystrophin [29].

Missense mutations result in single-nucleotide substitutions and are typically well tolerated, especially if within the dystrophin rod–encoding region of the gene. However, missense mutations can occur within vital gene regions such as splice sites, promoter regions, or within the cysteine-rich encoding region; these mutations are of greater consequence [30].

MODERN MANAGEMENT AND TREATMENT IN THE ERA OF STEROIDS AND BEYOND

The natural history of DMD before and after the introduction of steroids is shown in Fig. 3. Before treatment in the 1960s, loss of ambulation occurred in many boys by 9 to 10 years of age, and the mean survival age was 17.7 years. The introduction of surgical management of scoliosis and noninvasive ventilation did not alter motor function but significantly lengthened survival to a mean age of 27.9 years. Contemporary treatment that included the addition of corticosteroid treatment and improved cardiac management beginning in the 1980s lengthened the time of ambulation by 2 to 3 years and extended survival into the third decade. Prospective data from The Cooperative International Neuromuscular Research Group support continued corticosteroid treatment across the life span, even after the loss of ambulation [31].

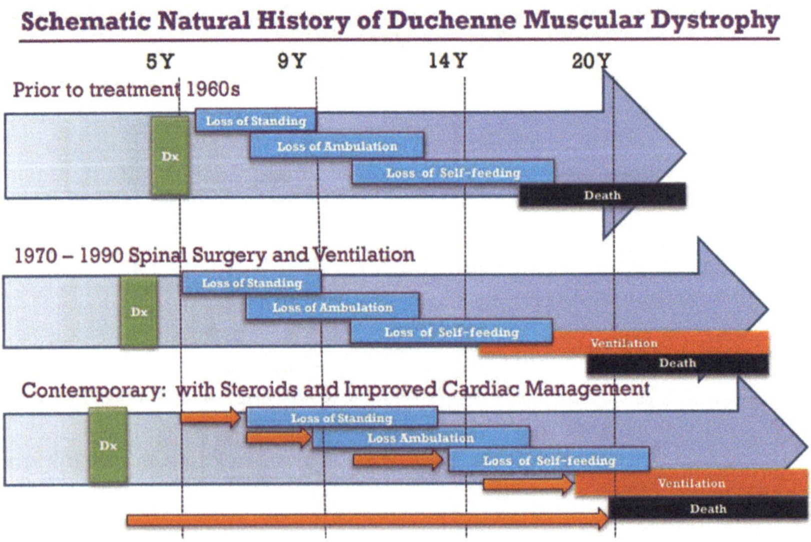

Fig. 3. Natural history of DMD. (*Top arrow*) 1960s: before treatment. (*Middle arrow*) 1970 to 1990: spinal surgery and ventilation added. (*Bottom arrow*) 1980 to present: steroid and cardiac management. Top arrow from McDonald C. Natural history of DMD/BMD: What is clinically meaningful? Oral presentation at The Cooperative International Neuromuscular Research Group; June, 2013; London, UK; middle and bottom arrows from McDonald CM, Henricson EK, Abresch RT, et al. The cooperative international neuromuscular research group Duchenne natural history study–a longitudinal investigation in the era of glucocorticoid therapy: design of protocol and the methods used. Muscle & Nerve 2013 July; 48(1):32–54; with permission.

Progressive functional motor decline begins in most boys by about 6 to 7 years of age. Coincident with a progressive decline, there is progressive multisystem involvement requiring multispecialty care. Because management only becomes more complicated with advancing age, early referral to a neurologist, physiatrist, or to an MCC is advised. MCCs are able to provide direct services by care center staff in attendance or by prompt referral to specialists not regularly present in the care center setting. This management approach has led to improved survival rates [32].

DMD care considerations published in 2018 [33–35] include management strategies in the following areas. The appropriate health care professionals who should be in attendance are indicated:

1. Neuromuscular management
   - Neurologist or physiatrist: establish diagnosis, monitor disease trajectory, steroid treatment management, Eteplirsen treatment of those eligible, keep abreast of on-going clinical trials, carrier detection
2. Respiratory
   - Pediatric pulmonologist: basic pulmonary function tests (mainly forced vital capacity), advise on use of noninvasive respiratory support (cough assist, mask ventilation)
3. Nutrition
   - Neuromuscular specialist and nutritionist: refer to a gastroenterologist for inadequate oral caloric intake
4. Cardiac
   - Pediatric cardiologist: interpret electrocardiogram and echocardiogram, cardiac MRI when necessary, prophylaxis and treatment of cardiomyopathy
5. Orthopedic
   - Pediatric orthopedist: monitor for scoliosis and joint contractures, ensure radiograph capability at the time of visit
6. Psychosocial
   - A social worker: provide and coordinate referrals and support to patients and families, psychological or psychiatric referral as needed
7. Rehabilitation
   - A physical therapist: assist with functional assessments, occupational and speech therapy availability, orthotics, and seating
8. Bone health
   - Neuromuscular specialist: monitor for adverse effects of limited weight bearing and steroid treatment, monitor vitamin D_3 intake, monitor for bone fragility by spine radiograph
9. Endocrinology
   - Endocrinologist: referral for management of complex bone health problems requiring intravenous (IV) bisphosphonate, monitoring of pubertal development as needed
10. Primary and emergency care settings
    - Overall health maintenance, including immunizations, emergency department for emergencies
11. Transitional care across the lifespan
    - Early planning and referral

A critical aspect of care that applies to almost every boy is steroid treatment. The exact age at which to begin steroids is not precisely defined, but a reasonable age range is 4 to 6 years, typically the plateau stage of DMD [33]. If the DMD phenotype is considered to be unusually severe, earlier treatment can be recommended. In contrast, if the phenotype is milder, parents might not be receptive to early treatment, and discussion of steroid treatment at each visit is necessary.

Whether to prescribe prednisone or prednisolone (0.75 mg/kg/d) or deflazacort (0.9 mg/kg/d) is controversial. Also, initiating treatment at a lower dose and gradually increasing it to the recommended maximum daily dose depending on response and tolerability is reasonable and often advised.

It is well established that steroids extend ambulation for an average duration of approximately 2 years or more compared with untreated boys [36]. Steroid treatment has also been shown to reduce the likelihood of scoliosis [37] that will require surgical intervention, and it prolongs upper limb and respiratory function for a variable period of time compared with untreated boys [38].

Deflazacort probably causes less weight gain and less behavior change than prednisone or prednisolone, but careful monitoring for all side effects is necessary for either steroid [38].

A clinical trial directly comparing prednisone with deflazacort is in progress with estimated completion in late 2019. It is hoped that the results of this trial will enable clinicians to make a more informed decision when prescribing either prednisone or deflazacort and also result in better dosing schedules.

Access to nongeneric deflazacort became a significant problem in the United States after the drug was granted US Food and Drug Administration (FDA) approval in February 2017. Thus far, deflazacort is manufactured by only 1 US pharmaceutical firm, and it can no longer be imported at a reasonable cost. Securing payment by patients' insurance carriers has been difficult.

TREATMENTS BEYOND STEROIDS

Therapies based on RNA modulation: antisense oligonucleotides

Eteplirsen is a phosphorodiamidate morpholino oligomer [39]. It is the only approved RNA modulating treatment that partially restores dystrophin expression. It is a synthetic strand of 30 morpholino rings, each serving as the backbone for a single nucleotide. The strand of 30 nucleotides attaches only to a specific complementary site on exon 51 of pre-mRNA near the exon 51–intron 51 junction. Eteplirsen is classified as an antisense oligonucleotide (ASO) because it attaches to the sense strand of pre-mRNA, hence antisense, and it is a short nucleotide strand, hence oligo, meaning few or small.

Eteplirsen partially restores dystrophin expression only in boys with frameshift DMD gene deletions that can be transformed to in-frame deletions by skipping (eliminating) exon 51 when pre-mRNA undergoes splicing. Amenable frameshift deletions must include exon 50 from the upstream direction or exon 52 downstream, and exon 51 must be present.

Removal of exon 51 expands the deletion size by an additional exon. However, the expanded deletion is transformed to an in-frame deletion because the total number of nucleotides deleted becomes a multiple of 3, as opposed to the original nucleotide number. The end result is an internally truncated but semi-functional dystrophin molecule produced from end to end that can be incorporated into the muscle protein cascade shown in Fig. 1. Even though truncated dystrophin production is limited, there is an increase in dystrophin-containing fibers that seems to be of some clinical benefit [40,41].

Accelerated approval was based on the surrogate end point of dystrophin production in treated boys, albeit in small quantities, but nevertheless reasonably likely to predict some degree of clinical benefit in an otherwise untreatable lethal disease [42]. Accelerated approval was granted with the understanding that the continuation of phase III studies is necessary to confirm the benefits after 2 additional years of treatment. Analysis of these data should soon be available.

Post–FDA eteplirsen approval studies showed an increase in dystrophin production after 180 weeks of treatment [43]. Additional studies showed slower rates of decline of respiratory function and use of upper extremities [44–46].

SYSTEMIC GENE TRANSFER (TRANSGENE THERAPY)

Mendell and colleagues [47] reported the results of 4 boys with DMD treated by single-dose IV delivery of microdystrophin (full-length gene is too large for viral vector) transgene with the MHCK7 promoter via an adeno-associated viral vector. The viral vector has high skeletal and cardiac muscle affinity, a low level of prior immunity, and it is not pathogenic in humans even though it easily enters muscle cells. The MHCK7 promoter drives gene expression selectively in skeletal and cardiac muscle. The microdystrophin transgene contains only the essential DMD gene components necessary for encoding a small but functional dystrophin protein. Boys ranged in age from 4 to 7 years, and had different mutation types between exons 18 and 58, no viral vector antibodies, below-average times on the 100-m walk test, CK levels greater than >1000 IU/L, and a stable steroid dose for at least 3 months before study entry. An additional daily steroid dose greater than their standard DMD dose was started 1 day before treatment and continued for about 30 days posttreatment [47].

Robust microdystrophin expression was shown by Western blot and by immunohistochemistry at 90 days. All clinical end points were met and CK levels decreased significantly. The duration of a single IV transgene infusion remains to be determined but, thus far, there is benefit up to 9 months. The transgene is found in muscle satellite cells, which should prolong the duration of action. Whether or not doses can be repeated will depend on immune responses.

This treatment is not mutation dependent and, if successful, will be available to most boys with DMD depending on the presence of viral antibody.

TREATMENTS IN DEVELOPMENT

- Two additional ASO skipping sites for exon 53 and 45 (in clinical trials)
- Second-generation ASOs with better skeletal and cardiac muscle penetration
- Ataluren for nonsense mutation readthrough
- Vamorolone, a dissociative steroid, with fewer side effects than glucocorticoids
- Nuclear factor-κB inhibition of inflammation and fibrosis
- B4GALNT2 (Beta-1,4-N-Acetyl-Galactosaminyltransferase 2) gene over-expression for modulation of muscle protein other than dystrophin

With the implementation of comprehensive DMD care consideration updated in 2018, further improvement in general health, motor function, quality of life, and survival is anticipated. Genetically based treatments, those approved and in clinical trials, should provide even more significant benefits.

Acknowledgments

The authors thank Elizabeth Kociolek for preparation of the text and figures for this article and Dr Jane Carver for critical review of the article.

Disclosure

Dr M. Gieron-Korthals does not have any commercial or financial conflicts of interest or any funding sources. Dr R. Fernandez served as a consultant for Sarepta's Regional Advisory Board. He does not have any financial or commercial conflicts of interest or funding sources.

References

[1] Koenig M, Hoffman EP, Bertelson CJ, et al. Complete cloning of the Duchenne muscular dystrophy (DMD) cDNA and preliminary genomic organization of the DMD gene in normal and affected individuals. Cell 1987;50(3):509–17.

[2] Jacobs PA, Hunt PA, Mayer M, et al. Duchenne muscular dystrophy (DMD) in a female with an X-autosome translocation: further evidence that the DMD locus is at Xp21. Am J Hum Genet 1981;33:513–8.

[3] Davies KE, Pearson PL, Harper PS, et al. Linkage analysis of two cloned DNA sequences flanking the Duchenne muscular dystrophy locus on the short arm of the human X chromosome. Nucleic Acids Res 1983;11(8):2303–12.

[4] Francke U, Ochs HD, de Martinville B, et al. Minor Xp21 chromosome deletion in a male associated with expression of Duchenne muscular dystrophy, chronic granulomatous disease, retinitis pigmentosa, and McLeod syndrome. Am J Hum Genet 1985;37(2):250–67.

[5] Hoffman EP, Brown RH Jr, Kunkel LM. Dystrophin: the protein product of the Duchenne muscular dystrophy locus. Cell 1987;51(6):919–28.

[6] Douglas AG, Wood MJ. Splicing therapy for neuromuscular disease. Mol Cell Neurosci 2013;56:169–85.

[7] Koenig M, Kunkel LM. Detailed analysis of the repeat domain of dystrophin reveals four potential hinge segments that may confer flexibility. J Biol Chem 1990;265(8):4560–6.

[8] Zhao J, Kodippili K, Yue Y, et al. Dystrophin contains multiple independent membrane-binding domains. Hum Mol Genet 2016;25:3647–53.

[9] Brenman JE, Chao DS, Xia H, et al. Nitric oxide synthase complexed with dystrophin and absent from skeletal muscle sarcolemma in Duchenne muscular dystrophy. Cell 1995;82: 743–52.

[10] Mokri B, Engel AG. Duchenne dystrophy: electron microscopic findings pointing to a basic or early abnormality in the plasma membrane of the muscle fiber. Neurology 1975;25: 1111–20.

[11] Bernasconi P, Di Blasi C, Mora M, et al. Transforming growth factor-beta1 and fibrosis in congenital muscular dystrophies. Neuromuscul Disord 1999;9:28–33.
[12] Murphy ME, Kehrer JP. Oxidative stress and muscular dystrophy. Chem Biol Interact 1989;69(2–3):101–73.
[13] Renault V, Piron-Hamelin G, Forestier C, et al. Skeletal muscle regeneration and the mitotic clock. Exp Gerontol 2000;35:711–9.
[14] Mendell JR, Shilling C, Leslie ND, et al. Evidence-based path to newborn screening for Duchenne muscular dystrophy. Ann Neurol 2012;71(3):304–13.
[15] Mirski KT, Crawford TO. Motor and cognitive delay in Duchenne muscular dystrophy: Implication for early diagnosis. J Pediatr 2014;165:1008–10.
[16] Connolly AM, Florence JM, Cradock MM, et al. One year outcome of boys with Duchenne muscular dystrophy using the Bayley-III scales of infant and toddler development. Pediatr Neurol 2014;50(6):557–63.
[17] Giliberto F, Radic CP, Luce L, et al. Symptomatic female carriers of Duchenne muscular dystrophy (DMD): genetic and clinical characterization. J Neurol Sci 2014;336:36–41.
[18] Mccaffrey T, Guglieri M, Murphy AP, et al. Cardiac involvement in female carriers of Duchenne or Becker muscular dystrophy. Muscle Nerve 2017;55:810–8.
[19] Grimm T, Kress W, Meng G, et al. Risk assessment and genetic counseling in families with Duchenne muscular dystrophy. Acta Myol 2012;31(3):179–83.
[20] Flanigan KM, Dunn DM, von Niederhausern A, et al. Mutational spectrum of DMD mutations in dystrophinopathy patients: application of modern diagnostic techniques to a large cohort. Hum Mutat 2009;30(12):1657–66.
[21] Wang Y, Yang Y, Liu J, et al. Whole dystrophin gene analysis by next-generation sequencing: a comprehensive genetic diagnosis of Duchenne and Becker muscular dystrophy. Mol Genet Genomics 2014;289(5):1013–21.
[22] Wei X, Dai Y, Yu P, et al. Targeted next-generation sequencing as a comprehensive test for patients with and female carriers of DMD/BMD: a multi-population diagnostic study. Eur J Hum Genet 2014;22(1):110–8.
[23] Klein CJ, Foroud TM. Neurology individualized medicine: When to use next-generation sequencing panels. Mayo Clin Proc 2017;9(22):292–305.
[24] Ankala A, da Silva C, Gualandi F, et al. A comprehensive genomic approach for neuromuscular diseases gives a high diagnostic yield. Ann Neurol 2015;77(2):206–14.
[25] Monaco AP, Bertelson CJ, Liechti-Gallati S, et al. An explanation for the phenotypic differences between patients bearing partial deletions of the DMD locus. Genomics 1988;2:90–5.
[26] Koenig M, Beggs AH, Moyer M, et al. The molecular basis for Duchenne versus Becker muscular dystrophy: correlation of severity with type of deletion. Am J Hum Genet 1989;45(4):498–506.
[27] Gurvich OL, Maiti B, Weiss RB, et al. DMD exon 1 truncating point mutations: amelioration of phenotype by alternative translation initiation in exon 6. Hum Mutat 2009;30:633–40.
[28] Bello L, Morgenroth LP, Gordish-Dressman H, et al. DMD genotypes and loss of ambulation in the CINRG Duchenne Natural History Study. Neurology 2016;87(4):401–9.
[29] Disset A, Bourgeois CF, Benmalek N, et al. An exon skipping-associated nonsense mutation in the dystrophin gene uncovers a complex interplay between multiple antagonistic splicing elements. Hum Mol Genet 2006;15:999–1013.
[30] Lenk U, Oexle K, Voit T, et al. A cysteine 3340 substitution in the dystroglycan-binding domain of dystrophin associated with Duchenne muscular dystrophy, mental retardation and absence of the ERG b-wave. Hum Mol Genet 1996;5:973–5.
[31] McDonald CM, Henricson EK, Abresch RT, et al. Long-term effects of glucocorticoids on function, quality of life, and survival in patients with Duchenne muscular dystrophy: a prospective cohort study. Lancet 2018;391(10119):451–461.
[32] Passamano L, Taglia A, Palladino A, et al. Improvement of survival in Duchenne muscular dystrophy: retrospective analysis of 835 patients. Acta Myol 2012;31:121–5.

[33] Birnkrant DJ, Bushby K, Bann CM, et al. Diagnosis and management of Duchenne muscular dystrophy, part 1: diagnosis, and neuromuscular, rehabilitation, endocrine, and gastrointestinal and nutritional management. Lancet Neurol 2018;17:251–67.
[34] Birnkrant DJ, Bushby K, Bann CM, et al. Diagnosis and management of Duchenne muscular dystrophy, part 2: respiratory, cardiac, bone health, and orthopaedic management. Lancet Neurol 2018;17:347–61.
[35] Birnkrant DJ, Bushby K, Bann CM, et al. DMD Care Considerations Working Group. Diagnosis and management of Duchenne muscular dystrophy, part 3: primary care, emergency management, psychosocial care, and transitions of care across the lifespan. Lancet Neurol 2018;17:445–55.
[36] Bello L, Gordish-Dressman H, Morgenroth LP, et al. Prednisone/prednisolone and deflazacort regimens in the CINRG Duchenne Natural History Study. Neurology 2015;85(12): 1048–55.
[37] Lebel DE, Corston JA, McAdam LC, et al. Glucocorticoid treatment for the prevention of scoliosis in children with Duchenne muscular dystrophy: long-term follow-up. J Bone Joint Surg Am 2013;95:1057–61.
[38] Gloss D, Moxley RT 3rd, Ashwal S, et al. Practice guideline update summary: Corticosteroid treatment of Duchenne muscular dystrophy: Report of the Guideline Development Subcommittee of the American Academy of Neurology. Neurology 2016;86(5):465–72.
[39] Kinali M, Arechavala-Gomeza V, Feng L, et al. Local restoration of dystrophin expression with the morpholino oligomer AVI-4658 in Duchenne muscular dystrophy: a single-blind, placebo-controlled, dose-escalation, proof-of-concept study [published correction appears in Lancet Neurol. 2009 Dec;8(12):1083]. Lancet Neurol 2009;8(10):918–28.
[40] Mendell JR, Rodino-Klapac LR, Sahenk Z, et al. Eteplirsen Study Group Eteplirsen for the treatment of Duchenne muscular dystrophy. Ann Neurol 2013;74:637–47.
[41] Mendell JR, Goemans N, Lowes LP, et al. Longitudinal effect of eteplirsen versus historical control on ambulation in Duchenne muscular dystrophy. Ann Neurol 2016;79:257–71.
[42] Woodcock J. FDA accelerated approval, eteplirsen, NDA 206488. 2016. Available at: https://parentprojectmd.org/wp-content/uploads/2018/04/Exondys51_FDA_Approval_Decision_Memo.pdf. Accessed November 25, 2019.
[43] Charleston JS, Schnell FJ, Dworzak J, et al. Eteplirsen treatment for Duchenne muscular dystrophy: Exon skipping and dystrophin production. Neurology 2018;90(24):e2146–54.
[44] Kinane TB, Mayer OH, Duda PW, et al. Long-term pulmonary function in Duchenne muscular dystrophy: comparison of eteplirsen-treated patients to natural history. J Neuromuscul Dis 2018;5(1):47–58.
[45] Khan N, Eliopoulos H, Han L, et al. Eteplirsen treatment attenuates respiratory decline in ambulatory and non-ambulatory patients with Duchenne muscular dystrophy. J Neuromuscul Dis 2019;6(2):213–25.
[46] Alfano LN, Charleston JS, Connolly AM, et al. Long-term treatment with eteplirsen in nonambulatory patients with Duchenne muscular dystrophy. Medicine (Baltimore) 2019;98(26): e15858.
[47] Mendell JR, Sahenk Z, Potter RA, et al. Systemic gene transfer with rAAVrh.74.MHCK7. micro-dystrophin in patients with DMD. Presented 12th Annual Neuromuscular Translational Research Conference. Newcastle-upon-Tyne, United Kingdom. April 4-5, 2019.